NURSING THE OPEN-HEART
SURGERY PATIENT

NURSING THE OPEN-HEART
SURGERY PATIENT

MARY JO ASPINALL, R.N., M.N.

Nursing Care Specialist

Long Beach Veterans
Administration Hospital

5929

McGRAW-HILL BOOK COMPANY

A BLAKISTON PUBLICATION

New York   St. Louis   San Francisco   Düsseldorf   Johannesburg
Kuala Lumpur   London   Mexico   Montreal   New Delhi   Panama
Rio de Janeiro   Singapore   Sydney   Toronto

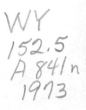

This book was set in Electra by Holmes Typography, Inc. The editors were Cathy L. Dilworth, Eva Marie Strock, and Sally Mobley; the designer was Michael A. Rogondino; and the production supervisor was Joan M. Oppenheimer. The drawings were done by Jean S. Stout.
The printer and binder was Kingsport Press, Inc.

NURSING THE OPEN-HEART SURGERY PATIENT

Library of Congress Cataloging in Publication Data

Aspinall, Mary Jo.
    Nursing the open-heart surgery patient.
    "A Blakiston publication."
    Bibliography: p.
    1. Cardiovascular disease nursing. 2. Surgical nursing. I. Title.
RC 674.A77   610.73'677   72-8364
ISBN 0-07-002410-3 (pbk)
ISBN 0-07-002411-1

1234567890   KPKP   79876543

To my husband, Bob, without whose help and encouragement this book would not have been written

CONTENTS

viii
Contents

Contents

Contents

FOREWORD

Challenges by Edith Olson, R.N.:[1]

I challenge you to keep knowledgeable, for as Thomas Huxley has said, "If a little knowledge is dangerous, where is the man who has so much as to be out of danger?"

Second, I challenge you to be actively involved in your Heart Association, for the choice is whether coming changes will be thrust upon health professions and community health agencies ill prepared to absorb or adapt to them, or whether organized health services and professions will seize their opportunities and influence the shape of the future. William James once said, "The great use of a life is to spend it on something that outlasts it."

Third, I challenge you to dream and to form your dreams into ideas and plans of action, for as Sir Joshua Reynolds has said, "The mind is but a barren soil—a soil which is soon exhausted, and will bear no crop, unless it be continually fertilized and enriched...."

And last, I challenge you to have faith in your dreams, for, according to the poet, Sir Rabindranath Tagore, "Faith is the bird that feels the light and sings when the dawn is still dark."

[1]From an address by Edith Olson, R.N., Nursing Coordinator, Rochester Regional Medical Program, delivered to the Council on Cardiovascular Nursing at the 44th Scientific Sessions of the American Heart Association. Used by permission of Miss Olson and the American Heart Association.

PREFACE

The heart is the life organ of the body; if it malfunctions, the life of the individual is threatened both physically and emotionally. The person whose heart performs inadequately must cope with a drastic change in his life style. If he is unable to make the necessary psychological adjustment, he may become depressed, become excessively dependent, become a cardiac cripple, or exhibit other emotional problems.

The development of the heart-lung bypass machine for heart surgery, prosthetic valves, and, more recently, heart-transplant operations and coronary bypass grafts, have given a new hope to those who had been incapacitated by their condition.

Nursing the open-heart surgery patient is both a challenging and a rewarding experience. The nurse needs an extensive background of theoretical knowledge as a base for her nursing care. She must understand the operation of the machines that monitor the many parameters, recognize critical physiological changes, make interpretative judgments, and take necessary action. She needs to translate information supplied by the inhuman machines into humane nursing intervention that meets both psychological and physiological needs of the individual. Total individualized care for each patient must be a team effort in which the patient and his family are included as well as the nurse, surgeon, cardiologist, social worker, spiritual advisor, and psychiatrist or psychologist.

This reference book presents essential theoretical concepts along with their practical application in assessment, intervention, and evaluation of nursing care. It includes continuity of care from the preoperative period through the many possible postoperative problems to the patient's return to the community.

This book is primarily intended for the graduate nurse who is preparing to give nursing care to patients undergoing open-heart surgery. However, as nurse educators respond to the challenge to prepare more nurses for the increased number of intensive care units, they are including advanced clinical experience in the basic nursing program. Thus this book will be a valuable reference for those students who have mastered the basic material and are searching for an advanced book for their continuing educational growth.

Since nurses are prepared at different educational levels, a comprehensive treatment is included of the three most crucial areas for the open-heart surgery patient: fluid and electrolyte balance, adequate respiration, and adequate circulation. Included in each of these sections is a brief review of the basic physiology so that the nurse will understand the terminology used and the normal functioning of these vital areas. Normal functioning is disrupted by heart surgery involving a cardiopulmonary bypass, and it is important for the nurse to understand the alterations that occur. These changes are explained in a manner intelligible to nurses, and the major symptoms for accurate nursing assessment are enumerated. Much nursing activity is necessarily the communication of vital information to the doctor and the carrying out of the doctor's orders. However, each section also includes specific measures that are primarily the nurse's responsibility.

The second part of the book presents special problems that may occur following open-heart surgery. The nurse should be aware of all these problems, although not all require specific nursing intervention. The role of the nurse is the focal point in the discussion of the major nursing problems of pain, reaction to stress, and role modification.

The appendixes contain concise but readily usable information on the surgical correction of heart defects; the major cardiac drugs; guidelines for some nursing procedures, with the rationale for the action; a sample of a nursing care plan; and a flow sheet for recording nursing observations.

The author's purpose in writing this book is twofold: to assist the nurse practitioner to render skillful nursing care to the patient with open-heart surgery, and to encourage the nurse researcher to join the author in exploring, testing, and evaluating new approaches to that nursing care that will make a contribution to the science of nursing.

The author is indebted to the following members of the staff of Long Beach Veterans Administration Hospital: Dr. Edward A.

Stemmer, Chief of Surgery, for his critical reading of the manuscript; Dr. Marvin A. Kaplan, Chief of Cardiology, for his assistance with interpretation of EKG strips; Timothy Dodge, Chief, Medical Illustration Section, and Ricardo Lopez, for photographic services; E. de Borra, Chief Nurse, and D. Atkins for their encouragement; and the nurses in the Surgical Intensive Care Unit, whose questions sparked the writing of this book and whose interest and concern saw it through to completion.

Mary Jo Aspinall

INTRODUCTION

1

The nursing care a hospitalized patient receives is determined to a great extent by the philosophy of the nursing service of the individual hospital. The philosophy of the author and of the surgical nursing service of the hospital in which she is employed is based on the premise that every patient has the right to physical, emotional, spiritual, and social well-being. Therefore the primary goal of the nursing service is to accept each patient and to develop his capabilities for maximum functioning as an individual, as a member of his family, and as a member of his community.

The individual nurse must have the capacity to show herself through personal and professional involvement in human existence. She must be capable of creative, independent thinking and sound judgments based on knowledge, understanding, and application of scientific principles.

This philosophy is contingent upon the basic premise of continuing personal and professional growth of each member of the nursing service. To implement this philosophy the major objectives of the nursing service are:

To provide safety for both patients and personnel by continuing awareness of factors that impede the normal therapeutic process and contribute to a hazardous environment.

To provide physical and emotional preoperative preparation by identifying individual needs and planning appropriate nurse intervention with consideration of semantic, cultural, and cognitive variables.

To provide close observation with the assistance of electronic monitors, to make interpretative judgments, and to render skillful nursing care to minimize the incidence of postoperative complications.

To provide a therapeutic environment that will encourage the patient's maximum involvement in his care, bolster his self-esteem, and help him to integrate the awareness of his surgical procedure into his self-concept.

To recognize the impact of illness and hospitalization on the patient, his family, and the community by planning with other disciplines to modify his environment as necessary following discharge to assure his maintained or continued progress.

To provide a learning environment that will contribute to the maximum development and utilization of each member of the nursing service.

To promote an administrative environment that is conducive to effective guidance and counseling, recognition of leadership potential, and job satisfaction.

To promote a progressive environment of continuing evaluation toward the improvement of the quality of nursing care and supervisory practice.

PREOPERATIVE PERIOD

2

The preoperative preparation of the patient is a vital factor in his response to surgery and his postoperative course. The patient who experiences a therapeutic environment in which both his emotional and physical needs are met is much better equipped to withstand the stress of the surgical procedure. A therapeutic environment is one that meets the needs of the individual patient, accepts the behavior of the patient, controls undesirable stimuli, helps the patient retain a sense of dignity and importance as a person, and promotes his understanding of the purposes and processes of his care.

DIAGNOSTIC PROCEDURES

Much of the patient's time in the preoperative period is spent in various diagnostic procedures. Since the patient encounters many new people during this period and laboratories and diagnostic departments tend to have rather rigid rules and restrictions for their effective functioning, the nurse needs to be skillful in coordinating the many activities and in supplying the element of human warmth and concern as well as information regarding the various tests. The usual diagnostic measures include the following:

1 *History.* This is taken in great detail and includes the presence, time of onset, and severity of the cardinal symptoms of heart disease: dyspnea, anginal pain, fatigue, palpitation, edema, and dizziness or syncope. The history also includes the presence of other physical conditions that might complicate surgery, such as hypertension, blood dyscrasias and clotting defects, chronic pulmonary disease, adrenal insufficiency, recent infections, and such conditions that affect the electrolyte balance as diabetes, chronic renal disease, and diarrhea. Finally, any drug allergies the patient has and all drugs he is presently taking, especially digitalis, anticonvulsants (for example, dilantin), diuretics, vasodialators, and anticoagulants are recorded.

2 *Laboratory examination.* This includes a complete blood count, electrolyte studies, arterial blood-gas determinations, serial blood cultures, if indicated, and a culture of any suspected possible foci of infection.

3 *Physical examination.* A physical examination includes noting the patient's general appearance (color, distension of carotid arteries, and character of venous waves in the neck when the bed is elevated 45°); peripheral pulse rate, rhythm, quality, and contour; and examination of the heart with a stethoscope, and palpation and visual inspection.

4 *Electrocardiographic examination.* This may include, in addition to the standard 12-lead EKG, an apex cardiogram (of the motion of the apex of the heart) to help determine the presence of mitral valve disease or mitral regurgitation.

5 *Radiologic examination of the chest.* This shows the position and size of the heart and aortic arch, the degree of vascularity of the lungs and whether the anterior or posterior part of the ventricle is greatly enlarged. Abnormalities in size may be due to an aneurysm or the effect of alterations in the flow of blood. It is important to compare chest films with previous films for changes.

6 *Special examinations.* Among the special examinations are pulmonary function tests; phonocardiograms to record murmurs and sounds, which are helpful in aortic stenosis or in detecting problems with previous prosthetic valve implants; brachial artery pressure curves which are made with a needle in the brachial

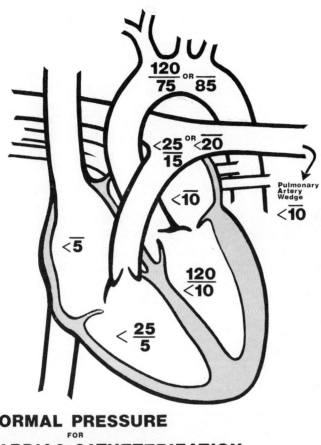

$$\frac{120}{75} \text{ OR } \frac{}{85}$$

$$\frac{<25}{15} \text{ OR } <\overline{20}$$

$<\overline{10}$

Pulmonary Artery Wedge

$<\overline{10}$

$<\overline{5}$

$$\frac{120}{<10}$$

$$< \frac{25}{5}$$

NORMAL PRESSURE
FOR
CARDIAC CATHETERIZATION

FIGURE 2–1 Schematic representation of the normal systolic, diastolic, and mean pressures in the heart chambers and major vessels. A properly obtained pulmonary artery wedge pressure corresponds to the pulmonary venous and left atrial pressure.

artery (this can be done as a separate procedure or as a part of cardiac catheterization); and cardiac catheterization and angiography, which is done to elucidate a difficult diagnosis. According to Dr. Swan [1],[1] information obtained from the procedure includes:

(a) Quantitative determination of cardiac output.

[1]Numbers in brackets indicate bibliographical references at the end of the book.

(b) Detection, localization, and quantification of abnormal intra- and extracardiac shunts.

(c) Measurement of intracardiac and great vessel pressure. Long-standing pulmonary congestion gives pulmonary hypertension, which complicates any surgical procedure (Fig. 2–1).

(d) Visualization of the size of the cardiac chambers and great vessels by angiocardiography to help detect dilatation or stenosis of the great vessels (Fig. 2–2).

(e) Cinecardioangiography (films taken at 60 frames per second to show movement of structures and contrast media) is used to observe the ventricle continuously over a period of time to determine its function. A mild degree of aortic regurgitation is best detected by injection of radiopaque contrast material into the ascending aorta just above the aortic valve.

A cooperative study by 16 laboratories over a 2-year period demonstrated that cardiac catheterization is attended by a significant hazard. Major complications occurred in 3.6 percent of the patients, with a mortality rate of 0.44 percent. However, the greatest majority of deaths occurred in the seriously ill infant [2]. The nature of the complications included:

1 Ventricular tachycardia and ventricular fibrillation—other arrhythmias occurred, but were not included as major complications.

2 Perforation of great vessels or the heart.

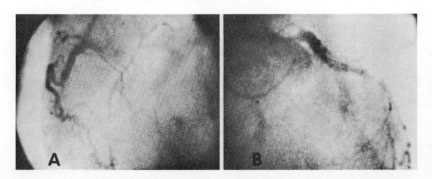

FIGURE 2–2   Coronary arteriography of the right coronary artery (A) and the left main coronary artery (B) of a 56-year-old man who had suffered myocardial infarction. Complete obstruction of the right coronary artery and the main anterior descending trunk of the left main coronary artery is demonstrated. *(From F. M. Sones, Jr., Cine Coronary Arteriography, in J. W. Hurst and R. B. Logue (eds.), "The Heart," McGraw-Hill Book Company, New York, 1970. Used by permission.)*

3 Emboli to brain, lungs, and major vessels, caused by displacement of embolic material at the time of cardiac catheterization.

4 Generalized cerebral dysfunction characterized by confusion, convulsions, or loss of consciousness—residual consequences were rare.

All patients should receive a test dose of the dye before the procedure to determine sensitivity. A frequent reaction to the dye is severe laryngeal spasm. Following the procedure, they should be watched for tachycardia, dyspnea, numbness of the extremities, and redness near the site of the injection, which can be caused by extravasation of the dye.

NURSING ASSESSMENT

The results of the diagnostic tests enable the nurse to assess the patient's physical condition, and her observation of the patient helps her to assess his psychological state. While the patient is involved with the various diagnostic procedures, the nurse observes his behavior and that of his family, and develops the kind of interpersonal relationship that permits the patient to explore his feelings without fear of judgment, punishment, or rejection. The nurse's demonstration of her acceptance of him is a prime factor in helping him identify and accept his own feelings. Through her interaction with him, she learns his perception of the nature of his disorder and his understanding of the surgical procedure and prognosis. She also identifies defense mechanisms he may be using to reduce the stress of the situation. The information she receives should be added to the initial assessment that is routinely made for all patients on admission. This expanded assessment is used as a basis for planning nursing intervention and patient education.

PREOPERATIVE PREPARATION

The patient needs to be prepared psychologically as well as physically for the surgery. Dr. Kaplan, in a study of 18 patients who had a mitral commissurotomy, found that the patients did not respond in any uniform manner to the surgery. The ways they adjusted to their physical improvement depended upon their total personality organizations and their life situations. Some patients immediately capitalized on their improved physical status, while others had utilized their illness as a means of adapting psychologically to their problems in life, and were therefore reluctant to give up their disability [3]. Thus for surgery to be effective it is important not only to relieve the underlying heart defect, but also any existing emotional problems.

Dr. Blurton, a psychologist at Long Beach Veterans Hospital, has successfully used group sessions with patients to help prepare them emotionally for the surgical procedure. The two major goals for the groups were (1) to supply knowledge about the procedure, which would reinforce the explanations given by the doctors and nurses, and (2) to help the patient arrive at a state of optimal readiness for surgery, in which he was neither phlegmatic and indifferent, nor fearful and rigid.

The group method has seemed more beneficial than individual sessions with the psychologist. Perhaps some factors responsible for its success are the benefit of identification with a group and the greater acceptance of the psychologist by a group than is usually found among individuals who attach a stigma to consulting a "shrink." The group identification decreases the feeling of loneliness, isolation, and concentration on oneself. The responsibility that patients feel toward other members of the group was often demonstrated in their eagerness to be transferred from the intensive care unit back to their cardiology ward so they could attend the scheduled meeting to reassure another patient scheduled for surgery.

NURSING INTERVENTION

Nursing Care

The main aspects of the nurse's role in the preoperative preparation of the patient include nursing care and patient education, based on the assessment of the patient's needs. The nurse can provide good care by following these nine guidelines:

- Ensure adequate rest by proper spacing of procedures and activities. If cardiac status necessitates complete bed rest, heparinization may be indicated to prevent formation of blood clots.
- Weigh the patient daily for early detection of fluid retention.
- Take the vital signs (including temperature and apical pulse rate) twice a day.
- Keep the patient on a low-sodium–low-cholesterol diet.
- Give the patient good skin care, including prompt treatment of acne or any other skin problem. Daily bathing with Phisohex or

other bactericidal soap is usually recommended, in spite of the current controversy over hexachlorophene. Avoid salt substitutes containing iodine because they may cause a skin problem. Encourage cotton pajamas rather than nylon in warm weather.

- Observe the patient closely for the presence of any infection.

- Administer medicine to control apprehension. Diazepam (Valium) is generally the best drug for mild to moderate apprehension. Any monamine oxidase (MAO) inhibitor drug is stopped at least 12 hr before surgery when Innovar is used for the anesthetic agent since it potentiates the action of Innovar. (MAO is an enzymatic preparation that inactivates toxic amines. Drugs like Marplan, Niamid, and Parnate are MAO inhibitors and cause an elevation in norepinephrine and serotonin levels.)

- Arrange for a clergyman, priest, or other spiritual advisor to bolster the patient's spirits during the preoperative period and prepare him spiritually and emotionally for surgery. The patient's social worker can help with monetary fears and the care of other family members while the patient is hospitalized.

- Stop all anticoagulants, digitalis, and diuretics 24 hr before surgery. Any beta-adrenergic blocking drug such as propanolol (Inderal) should be discontinued 3 weeks before surgery.

Patient Education

The nurse should plan an individualized program of teaching for the patient and his family, based on the present knowledge and on what the patient wants to know. Since in most hospitals patients receive their diagnostic work in a cardiology ward and then go to the intensive care unit after surgery, the responsibility for the preoperative teaching is usually shared by the nurses in these units. A transfer conference before surgery with the patient present gives an opportunity for the patient to get acquainted with the nurses who will be caring for him after surgery, and assures him that the nurses have heard and will respond to his requests. An example of a patient's request is that he be allowed to wear his glasses as soon as he is awake since they contain his hearing aid. The basic teaching given should include what to expect during the immediate preoperative and postoperative period. The patient should be told the routine aspects of the procedure, such as the preoperative skin preparation and shower, enema, and intravenous infusion, as well as the postoperative use of a respirator with an endotracheal tube or tracheostomy, Foley catheter, intravenous, EKG monitoring, chest drainage, and hypothermia. The depth of information given depends on the patient's desire to know (Fig. 2–3). A few patients prefer not to be told what will happen to them; therefore all details should be omitted for these patients. However, certain basic information must be given so they will realize that their situation post-operatively and the equipment being used is routine and does not mean that they are not doing well. Feedback information from the patient should be used to evaluate the effectiveness of the teaching. As Brambilla points out in her study of 20 open-heart surgery patients, the nurses' teaching plans should not only include material that the nurses think patients should know but should attempt also to answer the concerns and questions of the individual patient [4]. If the patient desires, he and his spouse should be allowed to visit the intensive care unit and see the equipment before his surgery. Seeing the person-

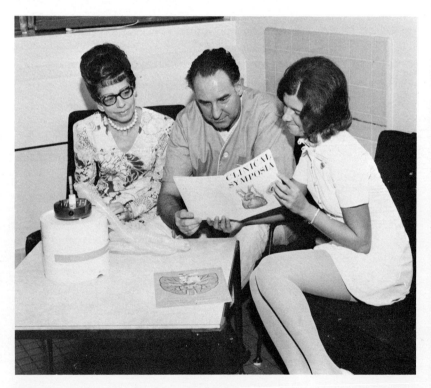

FIGURE 2–3 A conference with the patient and his wife gives the nurse an opportunity to tell the patient what to expect in the postoperative period and to answer any questions the patient may have. (Clinical Symposia containing drawings of the operative procedure used by permission of Ciba Pharmaceutical Company, Summit, N.J.)

nel working in the intensive care unit helps to reassure the patient that there will be competent persons to care for him and that they will be available when he needs them.

The patient should receive two or three intermittent positive-pressure breathing (IPPB) treatments with the same type of respirator he will be using in the postoperative period. The nurse should stress the importance of deep breathing and coughing, and provide practice periods for the patient during the preoperative period so he can become familiar with the techniques. Abdominal-diaphragmatic breathing is helpful because it increases the expansion of the lungs and helps the patient to exhale carbon dioxide more completely. The main aspects of this method of breathing should be demonstrated to the patient:

1   The nurse should instruct the patient to inhale quietly through the nose while using the diaphragmatic muscles to balloon out the upper abdomen.

2   The patient should then exhale through the mouth while flattening the abdomen. Exhalation should be continued until the abdomen has become "sunken-in."

3   After three to four deep breaths are taken by this method, instruct the patient to cough at the end of expiration. Adequate practice preoperatively has been found to result in more effective and productive coughing postoperatively.

The nurse should also emphasize the importance of exercises of the extremities (especially the lower extremities) to prevent venous stasis. Exercises that the patient should become familiar with preoperatively are alternating dorsiflexion and hyperextension of the feet and alternating flexion of the knee and thigh.

The patient should be encouraged to stop smoking. Some surgeons like to have smoking stopped for 3 weeks prior to surgery to reduce pulmonary insufficiency [5]. All patients should stop smoking at least 48 hr before surgery since catecholamines are increased by smoking. In the Framingham study of patients with myocardial infarction, the incidence of ventricular fibrillation was three times greater for patients who had smoked during the previous 48 hr [6]. Although no study has been made on postoperative patients, many physicians believe that results would be similar.

The patient and his family need to be thoroughly oriented to the hospital policy regarding visiting in the intensive care unit and usual length of stay. They also need to know that many patients experience a transient period of confusion in which they may misinterpret conversation or see objects that are not actually present. When they are prepared in advance for this occurrence, the patient speaks more openly when he experiences auditory or visual hallucinations and he is easier to reorient to reality.

THE OPEN-HEART SURGICAL PROCEDURE

3

Heart surgery is performed to correct anatomical abnormalities, repair or replace valvular defects, excise a ventricular aneurysm or akinetic area, or to improve the blood supply to the myocardium (a chart of the major heart defects and their surgical correction is Appendix A). Some surgical procedures can be done without artificial ventilation and circulation, but most procedures require either partial or total cardiopulmonary bypass. In partial bypass (or left heart bypass), the blood is drained from the left atrium and left ventricle and then returned by a pulsatile pump or a roller pump to the common femoral artery or the descending aorta. This procedure does not interrupt the pulmonary circulation.

In total cardiopulmonary bypass, a heart-lung machine that takes the responsibility for both oxygenation and circulation of the blood is used.

THE INCISION

A midline sternotomy incision is used for most surgical procedures, although an anterolateral thoracotomy with rib resection is used for a few procedures. A median sternotomy gives the best exposure and access to the heart without having to enter the pleural spaces, but it has a cosmetic disadvantage in that it frequently heals with a keloid and a broad scar [7]. After the chest wall is opened, the pericardium is opened to expose the heart. The patient is usually heparinized at this time using 9000 units of heparin per square meter of body surface or 300 units of heparin per kilogram.

THE CANNULATION

Cannulas are placed in the blood vessels to divert blood from the heart to the bypass machine and then to return blood to the patient. Arterial cannulation is accomplished by placing a cannula in the ascending aorta, the femoral artery, or the right external iliac artery. The arterial cannula is attached to the arterial line of the pump oxygenator. Venous cannulation is accomplished by placing cannulas in the inferior and superior venae cavae via the atrial appendage or through two openings in the right atrium. They are attached to the venous line of the pump oxygenator, and a partial bypass is started. A vent is usually introduced through the apex of the left ventricle or the left atrium and connected to the pump to aspirate intracardiac blood and maintain decompression (Fig. 3–1). It has been found that the fibrillating or asystolic heart is susceptible to irreversible damage from distension [8]. Frequently one of the suction lines is connected to a "thumbtack needle" vent that is placed in the ascending aorta for continuous evacuation of air bubbles or foam.

THE PERFUSION

The cardiopulmonary bypass machine is composed of a mechanical pump that simulates the pumping action of the left ventricle and an oxygenator that simulates the function of the lungs by creating a blood-gas interface for the exchange of gas (Fig. 3–2 and 3–3). Most pumps function by compressing a segment of tubing against a template. There are many types of oxygenators. The usual method of oxygenation employs thin sheets of plastic or rotating disks over which the blood becomes thinly filmed and then oxygenated as it is exposed to the atmosphere in the oxygenator chamber. Some oxygenators bubble the oxygen mixture from the bottom of a long column of blood in a chamber. The blood is foamy when it reaches the top of the chamber and is defoamed by passing over steel wool

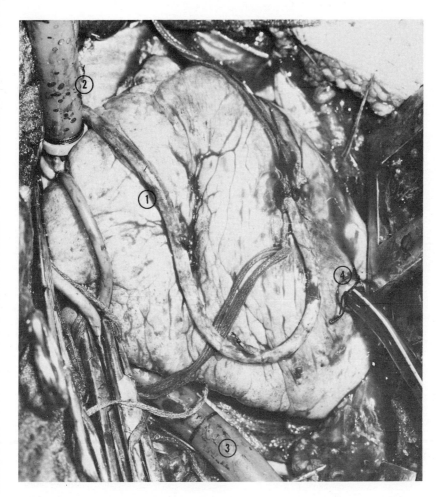

FIGURE 3-1   AORTOCORONARY BYPASS GRAFT SURGERY   (1) Saphenous vein graft from aorta to anterior descending branch of left coronary artery with an end to side anastomosis. (2) Cannula in superior vena cava. (3) Cannula in inferior vena cava. (4) Vent in left ventricle.

or a polypropylene mesh with a silicone antifoam compound on its surface. The perfusion is begun by sucking the venous blood into a reservoir connected to the oxygenator and concurrently returning the perfusate in the machine to the patient via the arterial cannula (Fig. 3-4). The perfusion is usually maintained at a rate of 2.2 to 2.4 l/min. per square meter of body surface.

  The gas used is usually oxygen, with 2 to 5 percent carbon

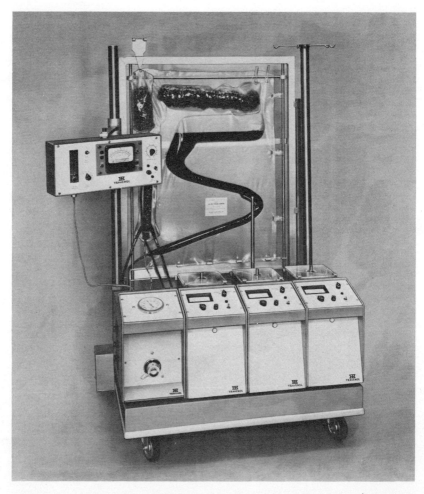

FIGURE 3-2 The Travenol heart-lung bypass machine utilizes a soft plastic unit with a heat reservoir. Oxygen is bubbled through the column of blood and then the blood is passed through a coated steel wool defoaming apparatus before return to the patient. *(Photograph courtesy of Artificial Organs Division, Travenol Laboratories, Morton Grove, Ill.)*

dioxide and a flow rate of 12 l/min. In earlier procedures, 100 percent oxygen was used, but it has been found that in all except very short procedures, excessively blowing off the carbon dioxide aggravates the metabolic acidosis because it reduces the formation of the bicarbonate base and decreases the body's ability to manage the excess acids being formed [9].

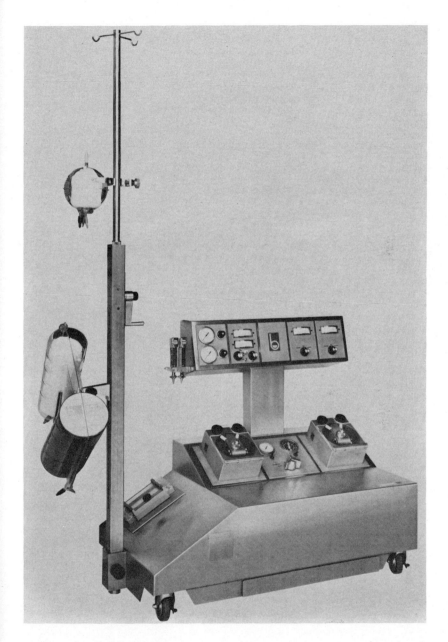

FIGURE 3–3 THE BENTLY TEMPTROL OXYGENATOR AND PUMP SYSTEM CONSOLE The bubble-type oxygenator has a hard shell and an integral heat exchanger. A polypropylene mesh coated with a silicone antifoaming compound is utilized to break up the bubbles. *(Photograph courtesy of Bentley Laboratories, Santa Ana, Calif.)*

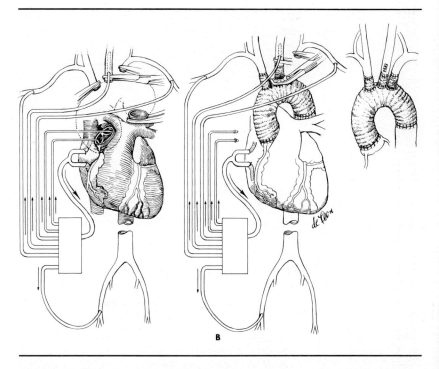

B

FIGURE 3–4 Diagram showing use of the cardiopulmonary bypass for graft replacement of an aneurysm of the aortic arch. Cannulae in the inferior and superior venae cavae divert the blood into the oxygenator and then the blood is returned to the femoral and carotid arteries. *(From M. E. DeBakey and A. C. Beall, Jr., Surgical Treatment of Diseases of the Aorta and Major Arteries, in J. W. Hurst and R. B. Logue (eds), "The Heart," McGraw-Hill Book Company, New York, 1970. Used by permission.)*

Temperature control is accomplished in most cardiopulmonary bypass machines by the use of an integral heat exchanger. In all except very short procedures, the perfusate temperature is used to cool the patient during the start of perfusion to 30 to 32°c (86 to 90°F). Cooling the patient reduces the metabolic rate and thus the oxygen consumption of the tissues without appreciably altering oxygen transport and other metabolic processes [10]. Rewarming is begun toward the end of the procedure to allow the patient's temperature to return to normal by the end of the perfusion period [7].

Hemodilution is used with most bypass machines. The minimum amount necessary to prime the machines varies between 850 and 1200 ml. Some physicians use only electrolyte solution or 5 percent dextrose in water for priming the machines; others use a mixture of blood and electrolyte solution. The advantages of hemodilution are that less blood is needed and capillary flow is increased because of the reduced viscosity and reduced rouleaux formation. The incidence of kidney damage is also less [11]. Since the gas exchange effected in the tissues, as well as in the oxygenator, depends on the concentration of red cells in the perfusate, the patient's blood should not be diluted to the point that the oxygen-carrying capacity is inadequate [9]. Most physicians dilute the blood to 50 to 75 percent or to a hemoglobin between 7 and 10. All blood that is used is collected within 24 hr to prevent severe acidosis. Some physicians remove the lymphocytes from homologous blood prior to cardiopulmonary bypass to avoid a possible homograft reaction of the cells of one individual against those of another [11].

Excessive trauma to the red cells is avoided whenever possible to limit hemolysis. Blood cells are unstable when they come in contact with air. Gas exchange in the lung is accomplished across the alveolar membrane. Although the present oxygenators give less trauma than the earlier models, there is direct contact between the gases and the blood. Besides the problem of hemolysis, it has been found that serotonin is released during prolonged pump oxygenation when there is continued trauma to the solid elements of the blood. Serotonin is a vasoactive substance that increases the resistance in the pulmonary arteries [12].

Air embolism is also carefully avoided. When the aorta is unclamped and the ventricles contain blood and air and are contracting, the air can be ejected through the aortic valve. Several techniques for prevention are used, and all air is evacuated from the cardiac chambers before the various incisions of the heart are closed [7].

Mortality increases with pump runs longer than 2½ to 3 hr, so cardiac surgeons practice to make their actions as smooth and efficient as possible. If the heart was electrically fibrillated, it is defibrillated after the air is evacuated.

Discontinuance of the heart-lung bypass should be done over a period of several minutes by progressively reducing the venous flow. The venae cava cannulas are withdrawn one at a time and the left ventricular vent is removed and the stab wounds repaired. The patient's own circulation takes up blood from the extracorporeal circuit until a satisfactory venous and/or left atrial pressure is reestablished. Except for mitral valve surgical patients, the patient is usually transfused to overfill the vascular compartment. Early maintenance of blood volume at an augmented level is done to improve ventricular function and provide a reserve against hidden blood losses [7]. If the heart beat is effective, protamine sulfate in amounts 1½ times the dose of heparin is given intravenously to neutralize the heparin. The arterial cannula is removed and the artery repaired. Two drains are usually used: one is placed in the retrosternal area and the other is in the right chest, with both drains connected to an underwater drainage system.

The sternum is closed with parasternal sutures of wire. Plain catgut is usually used for the subcutaneous tissues and #0 Tycron for the linea alba. Skin is usually closed with interrupted sutures of nylon.

CARDIAC PUMP FAILURE

A few patients are unable to maintain an adequate cardiac output. They may be placed on a partial bypass that utilizes a pump to take over part of the work of pumping blood from the left ventricle. Isoproterenol is given simultaneously to improve the pumping action of the left ventricle, and the patient can sometimes then be successfully removed from bypass. If the patient's ventricle still does not maintain an adequate cardiac output, some method of providing assistance to the left ventricle is needed.

One means of providing assistance to the left ventricle has been tried extensively in patients with cardiogenic shock following myocardial infarction. The method utilizes intraaortic counterpulsation with a balloon placed in the thoracic aorta. The balloon is inflated with helium at the end of ventricular systole and is deflated just before systole, to provide alternate expansion and contraction of the aorta. Since it lowers the pressure against which the left ventricle must pump it results in a lower systolic pressure and an increased cardiac output [13, 14]. The major disadvantage for its use after heart surgery is that it requires heparinization.

A new method of pulsatile bypass without heparin has been used experimentally and looks promising. It utilizes left atrial (and sometimes ventricular) cannulation to remove blood from the heart and a pulsatile pump with porcine aortic valves driven by conpressed oxygen to return the blood to the aorta [15, 16]. The plastic cannulas, tubing, and connectors are coated with a nonthrombogenic polyurethane-polyvinyl-graphite coating to prevent clot formation. The pulsatile pump seems to be more effective than nonpulsatile methods for maintaining adequate tissue perfusion. Systemic circulation has been maintained at almost normal levels, although there is no active driving force through the pulmonary circulation except for right atrial contraction. To maintain an adequate pressure gradient for pulmonary flow, the pulmonary vascular pressure must be kept low. Since pulmonary vascular resistance increases in proportion to the inspiratory pressure, the inspiratory pressure should be maintained at 10 mm mercury. This requires monitoring the blood gases and respiratory rates, with the administration of sodium bicarbonate to counteract metabolic acidosis [16]. This pump has potential for support of failing circulation in the immediate postoperative period.

FLUIDS AND ELECTROLYTES

4

FUNDAMENTAL CONCEPT OF HOMEOSTASIS

In order for the cell to survive and function, there must be mechanisms that regulate its immediate fluid environment. *Homeostasis* is the term applied to the body mechanisms which attempt to maintain a state of equilibrium of its structures, both solid and fluid. It involves the shifting of body water between intracellular, intravascular, and interstitial compartments and alterations in the concentration of numerous solutes.

NORMAL FLUID DISTRIBUTION

In normal individuals with an average amount of body fat, the fluid constitutes about 60 percent of the body weight. (Since fat is essentially water-free, when the amount of fat is less, the percentage of body weight that is caused by fluid is greater.) In newborn infants, total body water is 75 percent of the weight. Females may have a slightly lower percentage of body weight from fluids than males.

The total body fluid is distributed in two main compartments: intracellular and extracellular. The intracellular compartment, consisting of fluid inside the cells, makes up 55 percent of the total body water. The extracellular compartment, which makes up 45 percent of the total body water, may be further subdivided into:

1 The intravascular compartment (plasma), which forms 8 percent of the body water.

2 The interstitial compartment, which makes up approximately 20 percent of the body water.

3 Transcellular fluids involved with glandular secretion; they form 2 percent of the body water.

4 Bone, connective tissue, and cartilage, which make up 15 percent of the body water.

The functional extracellular fluid volume (FECFV) is that contained in the intravascular and interstitial compartments, since it is the only extracellular fluid readily available for exchange [17].

FUNCTION OF BODY FLUIDS

A fluid medium is essential for all body processes. The fluids making up the internal body environment serve the individual cells and serve to unite all body cells so the activities of cells in one area affect the activities of all other cells within the body. The blood plasma absorbs and transports nourishment and carries waste products to the organs of elimination: the lungs, skin, and kidneys. The interstitial fluid is an intermediary transport medium between the blood plasma and the cells.

COMPOSITION OF BODY FLUIDS

The average blood volume is about 5 l in an adult weighing 70 kg. Blood cells form about 45 percent of the total blood volume; plasma makes up 55 percent.

Two types of solutes are present in body fluids: *nonelectrolytes* and *electrolytes*. The nonelectrolytes, such as dextrose, urea, and creatinine, do not ionize in water solutions. Electrolytes are compounds whose aqueous solution will conduct an electrical current. They dissociate in solution to form separate, electrically charged particles called *ions*. A positively charged ion is called a *cation*. Cations in the body fluid are Na^+, K^+, Ca^{++}, and Mg^{++}. A negatively charged ion is called an *anion*. Anions in the body are Cl⁻, HCO₃⁻, HPO₄⁻⁻, SO₄⁻⁻, protein, and organic acid. The total number of cationic charges of an electrolyte always equals the total number of anionic charges.

Electrolytes are measured in milliequivalents per liter. An equivalent weight of a substance is that weight which will combine with or replace one gram of hydrogen. The equivalent weight can be calculated by dividing the molecular weight of the substance in grams by its valence. A milliequivalent (mEq) is one-thousandth of an equivalent weight and is used to express concentration of electrolytes in body fluids since the quantity is small. Because any given number of milliequivalents of a cation such as potassium would combine with the same number of milliequivalents of an anion such as chloride, the use of milliequivalents as a measure of available anions and cations for combination is helpful.

The fluid in each body compartment has a distinctive electrolyte pattern. In the intracellular fluid, potassium is the major cation and phosphate and protein are the major anions. In the extracellular fluid, sodium is the main cation and chloride is the main anion. Thus most of the sodium is outside the cell, and most of the potassium is inside the cell. The main difference in the two extracellular compartments (interstitial and intravascular) is the larger concentration of the anion protein in the intravascular fluid.

HOMEOSTATIC MECHANISMS

Regulation of Fluid Tonicity

The intracellular and extracellular compartments are separated from each other by a cell membrane. Cell membranes are freely permeable to water and semipermeable to most electrolytes. The plasma proteins and other colloids do not readily pass through the capillary wall. The movement of water and electrolytes is mediated by the two processes of *diffusion* and *osmosis*. Diffusion is the movement of the molecules (solutes) within a solution from a region of greater concentration to that of a lesser concentration. Osmosis is the movement of the fluid (solvent) across the membrane from the compartment of lesser concentration to the compartment of greater concentration. The force created by the particles in solution that attracts fluid across the membrane is termed *osmotic pressure*.

The osmotic pressure of the extracellular fluid depends upon the ionic concentration. When electrolytes are below normal, tonicity is decreased and the osmotic force of the extracellular fluid declines in relation to the cellular osmotic force and the fluid enters the cells; conversely, when electrolyte concentration is high, tonicity is increased and fluid passes from the cells into the interstitial lymph spaces and plasma until equilibrium is established.

The heart generates pressure as it pumps blood through the closed circulatory system. This force is termed *hydrostatic* or *filtration pressure*. This force acts in the opposite direction to the pulling-in power of the plasma proteins. The balance of water between the intravascular compartment tissues is the result of an equilibrium between water passing out of the vascular system, caused by hydrostatic pressure created by the pumping action of the heart, and the water reentering the blood stream because of the osmotic pressure generated by the plasma proteins and the concentration of electrolytes. More water leaves the vascular system than reenters it. This fluid is drained by the lymphatic capillaries and is eventually returned to the circulation.

Osmolarity, which can be defined as the total solute concentration, is a method of expressing osmotic effect. An osmol is a unit of osmotic pressure. Values are given in milliosmols (mOs), 1/1,000 of an osmol, since it is more convenient. For univalent ions, the mOs value is the same as the milliequivalent value. For mulitvalent ions, the mOs value is determined by dividing the milliequivalent (mEq) value by the valence number.

Normal blood plasma is 290 mOs. Solutions are considered isotonic, hypertonic, or hypotonic in relation to plasma with milliosmol values significantly the same, above, or below 290. Some of the milliosmol values of solutions are:

Solution	Millosmol values
0.45% NaCl	155 (hypotonic)
5% dextrose in H_2O	250 (hypotonic)
Ringer's lactate	290 (isotonic)
5% dextrose 0.11 NaCl	310 (isotonic)
0.9% NaCl (normal saline)	310 (isotonic)
5% dextrose/0.45 NaCl	410 (hypertonic)
5% dextrose/0.9 NaCl	560 (hypertonic) (This is the sum of mOs in 5%

Regulation of Fluid Volume

Water balance is maintained by the kidneys, lungs, skin, and gastrointestinal (G.I.) tract. Usually 1000 to 1500 ml is lost every 24 hr from the kidneys, 1000 ml by insensible perspiration from the lungs and skin, and 200 ml from the G.I. tract. The control of the volume of water in the body is a complex integrated mechanism involving both osmosis and stretch receptors in the heart and blood vessels.

Hypervolemia results in stretching of the group of receptors located in the left atrium, inhibiting production of antidiuretic hormone (ADH) and resulting in diuresis. Hypovolemia causes the stretch receptors in the left atrium to relax, stimulating the production of ADH and resulting in fluid retention.

Many other mechanisms contribute to the control of blood volume such as the level of sodium, secretion of aldosterone and adrenocorticotropic hormone (ACTH), and blood pressure. These will be discussed in more detail in other sections.

Regulation of the Hydrogen-ion Concentration

The acidity of a solution is determined by the concentration of its hydrogen ions. Acidity is expressed by the symbol pH, which stands for the potential of hydrogen. Neutral solutions have a pH of approximately 7, acid solutions have a pH of less than 7, and basic solutions have a pH of 7 to 14. The normal pH of the blood is 7.4. Alterations in tissue activities with the resultant production of acids and, to a lesser extent, bases will temporarily affect the acid-base equilibrium of the blood. The body has the following methods for regulating the concentration of the hydrogen ion:

Buffer System

The major buffer of the blood is *hemoglobin*, which buffers the blood against the large volumes of carbon dioxide that it transports. Most of the CO_2 that results from the metabolic process diffuses into the red blood cell where the enzyme carbonic anhydrase speeds up the combination with water, resulting in the formation of carbonic acid. Carbonic acid dissociates to give hydrogen and bicarbonate ions. The hydrogen ion released as a product of carbonic acid dissociation is buffered by the hemoglobin within the red cell. Most of the bicarbonate ion left free in the cell diffuses out of the red blood cell, resulting in diffusion of other negatively charged ions, chiefly chloride ions, into the red blood cell. Thus bicarbonate shift results in a compensatory chloride shift.

When bicarbonate diffuses from the blood into the plasma, it forms a large part of the buffer system of the plasma, the *bicarbonate-carbonic acid system*, which is also called the *alkali reserve*. Phosphate also acts as a buffer although it is more important in the urine than in the plasma.

A buffer system is a solution of a weak acid and one of its salts; it is formed by neutralizing a stronger acid with a strong base. The weak acid ionizes less completely than the strong acid it replaces, so it does not release hydrogen ions as readily as the stronger acid, and the hydrogen-ion concentration is less—thus the acidity is less.

The pH of a buffered solution is based on the relative quantities of the acid and salt components of the buffer. The Henderson-Hasselbalch equation expresses this ratio of bicarbonate to carbonic acid as 20:1 when the pH is 7.4. Thus the bicarbonate-carbonic system maintains a normal ratio of sodium bicarbonate to carbonic acid of 20 to 1. When an acid stronger than carbonic acid (for example, hydrochloric acid) enters the blood, it ionizes to the hydrogen ion (H^+) and the appropriate anion (Cl^-). The anion combines with the sodium in the sodium bicarbonate to form a salt ($NaCl$). The hydrogen ion unites with the bicarbonate anion to form the weak carbonic acid H_2CO_3.

$$(H^+ + Cl^-) + (Na^+ + HCO^{3-}) = NaCl + H_2CO_3$$

Abnormalities in hydrogen-ion concentration may be caused by metabolic or respiratory disturbances. Metabolic alterations occur as a result of primary changes in the bicarbonate-ion concentration, resulting in metabolic acidosis or alkalosis. Metabolic acidosis results from a deficit of carbonate (HCO_3). In metabolic alkalosis there is an excess of carbonate that is often associated with a deficiency of chloride or chloride and potassium.

Respiratory Mechanisms

In order to maintain a suitable level of the bicarbonate anion in the blood plasma and thus control the level of the hydrogen ion, carbon dioxide must be excreted by the lungs. A high concentration of carbonic acid stimulates respiration, which results in a decreased plasma carbon dioxide level. A low concentration depresses respiration and results in an increase in plasma carbon dioxide. This balance depends on the ventilatory capacity of the lungs to remove

CO_2. In hyperventilation, excessive carbon dioxide may be exhaled, resulting in depletion of the plasma carbonic acid and the hydrogen ions. Respiratory alkalosis will then result. In hypoventilation, which is usually caused by interference with gaseous exchange, carbon dioxide, carbonic acid, and hydrogen ions accumulate, causing respiratory acidosis. This is a frequent complication during surgery. Respiratory acidosis and respiratory alkalosis will be discussed in more detail in a later section.

Renal Excretion

The kidney plays a part in controlling the hydrogen-ion concentration by selectively reabsorbing or rejecting both cations and anions. Although the kidney is able to excrete either an alkaline or an acid urine, the urine is usually acid (pH = 6). The lowest pH that can be achieved is 4.4. Phosphates are the main buffers of the urine. Maintenance of the normal hydrogen-ion concentration is accomplished by maintaining the serum bicarbonate between 26 and 28 mEq/liter and the excretion of excess hydrogen ions. In response to an increase in the acid in the blood, the kidneys excrete an acid urine that conserves the base by reabsorption of the bicarbonate, preventing a large drop in pH.

An example of the process of elimination of the hydrogen ion is the combining of ammonia with a hydrogen ion to form the ammonium ion. Thus each molecule of ammonia removes one hydrogen ion. Since ammonium ions can replace sodium or other cations in the urine, it allows for the excretion of "strong" anions without losing necessary cations.

ORGANS OF REGULATION OF FLUID AND ELECTROLYTE BALANCE (Fig. 4-1)

The Heart and Blood Vessels

These vessels regulate the formation of urine by their control of blood pressure. The effect of the hydrostatic pressure on osmosis has been discussed previously. Arterial blood pressure of at least 70 mm Hg is necessary for the formation of urine. However, adequate blood pressure does not assure normal urine flow.

The Kidney

In a normal individual who receives adequate quantities of fluid and electrolytes, the kidney selectively retains only what is needed

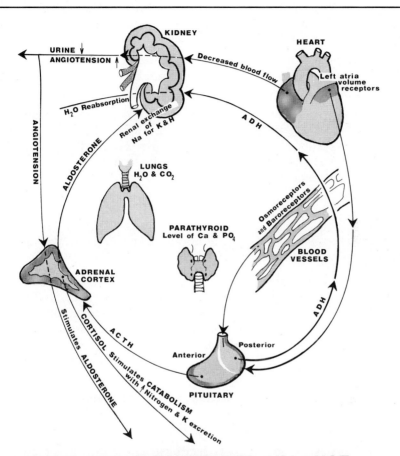

FLUID AND ELECTROLYTE BALANCE

FIGURE 4-1   The maintenance of homeostasis is a complex process involving mechanisms for regulating fluid volume, tonicity, and electrolyte levels.

for restoration and maintenance of homeostasis. In disease, this selective capacity is impaired.

The *renal tubules of the kidney* are responsible for:

1   *Active reabsorption.* In a 24-hr period, the kidneys produce about 180 l of glomerular filtrate. Of this amount seven-eights is reabsorbed through the proximal tubules, along with solutes. About 85 percent of the sodium is reabsorbed plus

some glucose, urea, and other substances. The kidney conserves potassium poorly, and potassium is mainly excreted, not reabsorbed. Chloride may be excreted with potassium.

2 *Secretory activity.* Ammonia and hydrogen are secreted from the distal tubule cells, and ion exchange follows, which is important in acid-base regulation.

3 *Concentration of the urine.* If the kidneys can concentrate adequately (up to specific gravity of 1.035), the urine output can be reduced to about 900 cc per 24 hr. If the kidney function is impaired, more water will be required to excrete the same amount of solute.

The Posterior Lobe of the Pituitary

This lobe secretes an antidiuretic hormone known as ADH. Among the factors responsible for ADH release are:

An increase in the osmotic pressure of the blood. This stimulates nerve receptors in the internal carotid arteries, and their impulses in turn cause release of ADH from the pituitary. When ADH is secreted, the distal convoluted and collecting tubules become more permeable to water molecules and more water is reabsorbed, which may restore the blood to normal concentrations.

Decreased body fluid volume, visceral manipulation, pain via somatic nerves, shock, and stress may also stimulate the release of ADH.

Conversely, a decrease of electrolyte concentration or an increase in body fluid volume suppresses the release of ADH and permits an excess output of dilute urine.

Although most authors feel the osmotic pressure is the main regulator of ADH secretion, Gauer and others believe the strongest stimuli to release of ADH are related to changes in the blood volume, with the sensing elements located in the blood vessels and heart, primarily in the left atrium and responding to changes in vessel and left atrial pressure [18].

The Anterior Lobe of the Pituitary

The anterior lobe secretes regulatory hormones for other endocrine glands called *tropic hormones.* One of the most important of these is the adrenocorticotropic hormone (ACTH), which stimulates the adrenal cortex to secrete its hormones. Elevated serum potassium concentration and numerous factors that accompany stress and injury liberate ACTH to stimulate aldosterone release.

The Adrenal Cortex

This organ secretes the mineralocorticoid *aldosterone,* which increases the reabsorption of sodium in the distal tubules. Aldosterone stimulates a potassium-sodium exchange system, raising the plasma sodium and lowering the plasma potassium. Some stimuli that increase the secretion of aldosterone are decreased blood pressure in certain branches of the internal carotid artery, decreased blood flow to the juxtaglomerular structures of the kidney, and increased secretion of ACTH following stress and injury.

The Parathyroid Glands

The parathyroid glands are stimulated to secrete their hormone when the blood calcium level falls. The parathyroid secretion regulates the extracellular concentration of calcium and phosphate ions by increasing the rate of release of calcium from the bones, enhancing its absorption from the intestine, and increasing the excretion of phosphorus and the absorption of calcium from the kidneys.

THE EFFECT OF OPEN-HEART SURGERY ON THE FLUID AND ELECTROLYTE BALANCE

Changes in the secretions of the pituitary and adrenal glands are a normal body response to trauma or any surgical procedure. In addition, the open-heart surgery patient may have unique alterations in electrolytes and fluids caused by the cardiopulmonary bypass procedure. In patients who have cardiac decompensation there is also a tendency to retain water and extracellular salt with an increased venous pressure in either the right or left atrium, or both [19].

The usual fluid and electrolyte pattern following open-heart surgery includes:

1   Increase in the level of free blood cortisol, which stimulates tissue catabolism with a resultant lysis of cell protoplasm and protein with a release of amino acids and cellular electrolytes, namely potassium, into the extracellular fluid.

2   Renal retention of water, sodium, chloride, and bicarbonate
with the excretion of potassium, and a resultant expansion
and dilution of the FECFV. Dilution of the FECFV lowers the
plasma osmolality and may result in hyponatremia, although
there is an excess of total body sodium.

3   Fluid diffuses from the intravascular space during and after
cardiopulmonary bypass. Part of the fluid is excreted by the
kidneys, and some passes into the interstitial compartment and
then gradually returns to the intravascular compartment. Rigid
curtailment of postoperative fluids is necessary to prevent
fluid volume overload and heart failure on the fourth or fifth
postoperative day as the perfusate reenters the intravascular
compartment [11].

GENERAL PRINCIPLES OF WATER AND ELECTROLYTE BALANCE MANAGEMENT

Preoperative Period

Prolonged fluid limitation and the use of cathartics and diuretics
before surgery may result in dehydration and deficits of electrolytes, red blood cells, and albumin. Any deficiency should be
replaced before surgery. Red cell volume, electrolytes, and fluid
are easily replaced. Albumin has an intravascular half-life of only
12 hr and is thus more difficult to replace. However, albumin is
essential for the maintenance of the colloid osmotic pressure of
the blood. It cannot be given rapidly to most patients since each
gram retains within, or attracts into, the vascular compartment
20 ml of water. Usually 2 or 3 units a day are given over a period of
several days before the surgical procedure. The weight should be
obtained daily, as a guide to be used on into the postoperative
period. The central venous pressure and hourly urine outputs are
other fluid volume guides that will be discussed in a later section.

Intraoperative Period

Blood loss during a surgical procedure is usually replaced to within
10 percent of the blood loss. The loss of functional extracellular
fluid volume (FECFV) during an operation is more difficult to
estimate than blood loss. Shires found that the extracellular fluid
lost is related to the extent of the surgical trauma rather than to the
volume of blood lost [20]. In extended operations where there is

aortic cross-clamping that involves much trauma and blood loss, a great deal of extracellular fluid may be lost. The replacement of the fluid deficit with fluid containing electrolytes, which is isotonic, such as Ringer's lactate, at a rate of at least 5 ml/kg/hr (300 ml/hr for a man of 150 lb) is recommended. A unit of albumin or plasma for each 2 liters of electrolyte solution is also recommended for provision of essential colloid to replace protein lost by exudate or transudate [17].

The management of fluid volume, blood, and electrolytes while the patient is on the heart-lung bypass machine is a complex procedure, with great differences of opinion. No attempt will be made to cover all the various approaches, but two methods will be briefly discussed.

One method of management is the use of as little blood as possible, allowing the hemoglobin to drop to 7, but adding sodium bicarbonate to combat acidosis resulting from low hemoglobin. Mannitol is also used to cause diuresis and raise the hemoglobin without the administration of blood. Another method of management is the physiological replacement of blood, fluids, and electrolytes. Although hemodilution is allowed while on the pump, blood is replaced as the patient is removed from the pump so the hemoglobin is no lower than 12.

Postoperative Period

Fluid Therapy

After open-heart surgery, the main objectives of parenteral fluid therapy are to:

- Maintain an effective circulating blood volume.
- Prevent the impairment of the colloid osmotic function of the blood that results when the serum albumin is low.
- Maintain a urine flow of at least 30 ml/hr to prevent tubular necrosis from precipitation of hemolyzed blood.
- Replace in volume fluid lost externally (including insensible loss) and internal translocations of FECFV into the cells. Fluid volume is usually held to 1500 ml for the first 24 hr after surgery and gradually increased. Additional fluid is administered if the physical symptoms and central venous pressure measurements indicate that the additional fluid load can be tolerated.

- Supply ascorbic acid (usually 300 mg/day) and multiple B vitamins.
- Maintain electrolytes within normal limits. Values considered normal at Long Beach Veterans Hospital are:

Sodium (Na)	135–145 mEq/l
Potassium (K)	3.5–5.0 mEq/l
Chloride (Cl)	95–105 mEq/l
Calcium (Ca)	9.0–11.5 Mg% or 4.3–5.3 mEq/l
Magnesium (Mg)	1.5–2.5 mEq/l
Phosphate (PO_4)	2.6–3.2 mEq/l
Bicarbonate (HCO_3)	24–31 mEq/l

Magnesium, phosphorous, and bicarbonate are often not measured (see chart at end of chapter).

Electrolytes

Sodium is the most important cation in maintaining the fluid balance. Surgeons are not in agreement on the administration or restriction of sodium for the open-heart surgery patient. The prevailing theory for the past several years has been that water and sodium are retained postoperatively primarily because of the endocrine mechanisms of ADH and aldosterone initiated in response to the stress of surgery. The logical application of this concept led to the postoperative use of parenteral solutions without sodium, or very low in sodium.

In recent years some physicians have begun to question whether salt and water retention were entirely the result of endocrine production or whether they were a reflection of a disorder of volume, composition, or distribution. Crandell [17] has hypothesized that following surgery increased ADH and aldosterone are released, resulting in water and sodium retention. With extensive surgery there is a translocation of extracellular fluid, chiefly an obligatory movement into the area of injury. With the relocation of functional extracellular fluid, transcapillary filling is less effective and the diminished blood volume leads to the release of more ADH and aldosterone. If the intravascular and extracellular fluid volumes are promptly replenished, this hormonal response can be lessened. Thus the usual postoperative renal conservation of sodium is felt to result from a contraction of the FECFV consequent to a sequestration of fluid in and around tissues traumatized by operation [21]. Therefore, most surgeons give 50 to 150 mEq of sodium on the operative and first postoperative day to provide the solute load necessary to overcome the antidiuretic stimulus. Some surgeons prefer to limit sodium and give mannitol, but sodium is probably more physiological [19].

Potassium is essential for normal cellular functioning, maintenance of acid-base balance, and electrical conduction in the heart muscle. Hypokalemia potentiates the action of digitalis and may result in digitalis toxicity. Since only 1 percent of the body potassium is outside the cell, the serum potassium is an insensitive indicator of cellular potassium. The serum potassium level is increased in acidosis as the hydrogen ion entering the cell replaces the potassium ion. It is decreased in alkalosis as potassium shifts back into the cells.

Surgery mobilizes considerable amounts of potassium with the breakdown of cells; therefore, a normal serum potassium was used in the past as an indication that no potassium needed to be administered for at least the first 24 hr after surgery. Studies made by Krohn demonstrated that metabolic alkalosis with large urinary losses of potassium occurred commonly after heart surgery. Patients with poor myocardium can lose 300 mEq of potassium in the urine every 24 hr [22]. Since patients do lose potassium, 40 to 80 mEq of potassium chloride is usually given daily postoperatively if the patient is excreting urine. Greater amounts may be given to replace heavy urinary losses of potassium. Sometimes all urine is saved for 24 hr determinations of potassium. If low protein is present with hypokalemia, the protein level has to be raised before the hypokalemia can be corrected, since with tissue breakdown potassium is rapidly excreted. The usual precaution in the administration of potassium is that no more than 20 mEq be given in one hour and that the administration be discontinued until the surgeon can reevaluate the situation for any of the following reasons:

1 A decrease in urine volume to less than 20 ml/hr for two consecutive hours

2 Elevation of serum creatinine

3 Elevation of blood urea nitrogen (BUN)

4 EKG changes indicative of hyperkalemia: biphasic wave, wide QRS, long PR interval, and peaked T wave

5 Serum potassium elevated above 6

Chloride level is not subject to much variation. Changes of the chloride ion concentration in the plasma follow those of sodium in most situations, with a dilutional hypochloremia accompanying a dilutional hyponatremia. A high level of adrenal corticosteroids may result in sodium retention with potassium and chloride loss. Hypochloremia may also be associated with a hypokalemic metabolic alkalosis. When chloride replacement is needed and the levels of sodium and potassium make it undesirable to give NaCl or KCL, lysine monohydrochloride is the preferred replacement therapy.

Approximately 90 percent of the body *calcium* is found in the form of calcium phosphate and calcium carbonate in the bone. When the serum calcium falls, the bones act as a ready source of calcium. Under normal body situations, the ionized portion of the serum calcium constitutes about 50 percent of the total blood calcium. Most nonionized calcium is bound to protein. Ionized calcium is necessary for blood coagulation, normal cardiac and skeletal muscle contractions, and nerve function. The parathyroid glands control the level of plasma calcium, but the level of the serum proteins and the pH of the extracellular fluid affect the percentage of ionized calcium. In the presence of low serum protein, low total calcium may yield a normal amount of ionized calcium.

When the extracellular fluid becomes acidic in reaction (metabolic acidosis) there is a shift of protein-bound calcium toward ionized calcium. This results in an increase in the percentage of ionized calcium and a decrease in the nonionized percentage of calcium. With metabolic alkalosis, the percentage of ionized calcium decreases, and the total calcium is unchanged. Thus a patient with a low serum calcium may have an adequate amount of ionized calcium if he is in metabolic acidosis. A rapid correction of the acidosis may result in symptoms of hypocalcemia because of the decrease in ionized calcium, therefore therapeutic management attempts to avoid rapid changes in the acid-base ratio that do not allow time for mobilization of calcium from the bones. A reciprocal relationship exists between the calcium and phosphorus ions (phosphate). As the level of phosphorus rises, calcium decreases.

Calcium has a synergistic action with digitalis. Digitalis toxicity may develop when the level of calcium increases. Calcium also antagonizes potassium. This antagonistic action is probably related to the need for phosphorus to move potassium in and out of the cell. Since increasing the calcium level decreases the phosphorus level, potassium movement is inhibited. Thus in general, when potassium is needed, calcium is not given.

Patients receiving large amounts of citrated blood may have a decrease in the level of ionized calcium since the citrate binds the free calcium. A few surgeons follow the practice of giving calcium with each third unit of blood to combat this tendency. If calcium is given, care must be exercised that it is never given into the same line as the blood since it will cause the blood to clot. Most surgeons do not give calcium except for symptons of calcium deficiency. Some symptons are:

1 Numbness and tingling of the nose, ears, fingertips, and toes, which progresses to muscle cramps and tetany.

2 An EKG picture that demonstrates a prolongation of the Q-T interval caused by the lengthening of the S-T segment.

3 Presence of Trousseau's sign, which can be elicited by grasping the patient's wrist so as to constrict the circulation for a few minutes. If his hand goes into a position of palmar flexion (carpopedal spasm), he probably has a serious calcium deficit.

4 Presence of Chvostek's sign, which can be elicited by tapping the patient's face lightly over the facial nerve (just below the temple). A calcium deficit is probably present if the facial muscles twitch.

5 A serum calcium below 4.3 mEq per liter, which needs to be carefully evaluated with the serum protein and pH.

Calcium gluconate is usually given for symptomatic hypocalcemia. Calcium chloride may be given for acute conditions since it ionizes faster.

Magnesium is mainly distributed within the cells. About 35 percent of it is bound to protein. Magnesium is essential for activation of enzymes necessary for mediation of the energy processes of the cell. The manifestations of deficiency are the same as those seen in hypocalcemia. Normally body stores of magnesium are sufficient to last for a month without replacement. The chronic alcoholic may have less magnesium reserve because of the lowered capacity of the liver to maintain a high cellular concentration of magnesium. If patients are on excessively prolonged intravenous therapy, usually 10 to 15 mEq of magnesium are added to the IV fluid daily.

Positive Nitrogen Balance

Intravenous therapy aims to provide sufficient calories to minimize ketosis and protein breakdown. Five percent dextrose solutions contain only 200 cal per liter. Since total daily parenteral intake is usually less than 3 liters, 5 percent dextrose solutions do not supply an adequate number of calories. Ideally patients are quickly progressed to oral intake. It has been found that excessive intravenous therapy after the seventh postoperative day when some oral intake and ambulation had not been achieved results in an increase in mortality [23].

If the patient is unable to progress to oral alimentation after a week, some surgeons feel that sufficient calories and protein to produce a positive nitrogen balance should be provided by the intravenous route. Proponents of this type of parenteral hyperalimentation believe that 50 cal/kg body weight/day (or 3500 cal for the average 70-kg man) is needed to provide a positive nitrogen balance because if not enough dextrose is given with the amino acids to supply the energy requirements, the amino acids will be utilized for energy instead of protein restoration [24]. Since sugars provide about 4 cal/gm, a 20 percent solution of glucose will provide 800 cal/l. Fifty percent glucose may also be given for more calories (2000 cal/l). Amino acid solutions such as 5 percent protein hydrolysate in 5 percent dextrose are usually mixed with an equal volume of hypertonic dextrose. One liter of amino acids supplies 50 gm protein and 50 gm glucose (total 400 cal). Insulin is usually given on a rainbow scale for urine sugar, but if the patient is not a diabetic, he will rarely need insulin after the first or second day of therapy. Remember that intravenously administered dextrose carries potassium from the extracellular fluid into the cells so additional potassium is usually given with high concentrations of dextrose. Because of the higher incidence of bacterial contamination in hypertonic glucose solutions, these solutions should be prepared under a laminar flow hood and stored in the refrigerator until used. Parenteral hyperalimentation should be administered by gradually increasing the amount of calories in increments of 1000 to 1500 cal per day until the amount necessary for positive nitrogen balance is reached. Ethyl alcohol is a good source of calories and is well tolerated. Fifty milliliters (50 gm) of 95 percent ethyl alcohol added to 1 liter of other IV fluid will supply an additional 350 cal and is not intoxicating when the rate of administration does not exceed 10 gm/hr for an adult.

Intravenous fat emulsions are sometimes used to provide calories, but their use has been restricted in the United States because of the development of fat emboli and the fat overloading syndrome for some patients. All hypertonic solutions of more than 750 mOs tonicity should be given in a large vein (preferably in the subclavian) with a Teflon catheter. They should also be given at a uniform rate over the 24-hr period. Hypertonic dextrose infusions may cause osmotic diuresis and result in cellular dehydration with a high concentration of all serum solutes. Thus electrolyte and the blood urea nitrogen concentration need to be checked frequently. If the patient is progressed to high protein tube feedings, enough water must be given to promote excretion and prevent cellular dehydration.

NURSING ASSESSMENT OF FLUID AND ELECTROLYTE BALANCE

Fluid Intake

Fluid intake needs to be accurately measured (see chart at end of chapter). The type of fluid needs to be recorded as well as the amount since albumin or fluid high in glucose or sodium may result in an osmotic shift of water and electrolytes from the interstitial space to the plasma. Intake of ice chips is best measured when two containers of the same size are filled with ice chips. One is given to the patient and the other is allowed to melt and is then measured and the amount recorded. All intake is totaled at least every 8 hr and compared with output.

Urine Monitoring

Urine should be checked for:

Output

Urine output is measured hourly. Output should be at least 30 cc/hr. The type of solute load given intravenously affects the urine output. For example, each 12.5 gm of mannitol given will result in excretion of approximately 135 ml of urine unless the kidney is not functioning. The relationship of blood pressure to urinary output has already been discussed. Usually a systolic pressure of 70 mm Hg is necessary for the kidneys to excrete urine. A urinometer is available to automate the output record, but most nurses have not found it to be helpful.

Specific Gravity

This is measured every 1 to 2 hr. A high specific gravity (1.030) usually indicates dehydration. Scanty urine with a low specific gravity is usually indicative of renal failure. Normal specific gravity is 1.015 to 1.025.

pH

The pH of urine is measured every 1 to 2 hr (Fig. 4–2). Normal pH is 6. The urine pH reflects the serum pH except in hypokalemic alkalosis when the urine pH is acid (termed *paradoxical aciduria*).

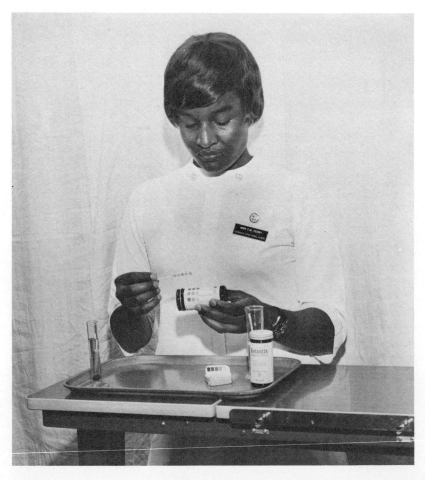

FIGURE 4–2 Measurement of the pH of the urine can be done quickly by the comparison of the color change on commercially available indicator sticks.

Electrolyte Concentrations of Sodium and Potassium

Determinations of these concentrations are helpful in confirming the presence or absence of deficits in total body sodium and potassium. The daily urinary losses of potassium are particularly helpful in determining the need for potassium.

Other Fluid Losses

Such fluid losses as chest drainage and nasogastric tube drainage are also carefully recorded. If there is significant drainage, dressings should be weighed. Every kilogram of increase in weight of wet dressings over dry dressings represents an output of 1000 ml.

Weight

Weight is usually obtained daily at a specific time. Bed scales are used, and variations in weight from linen are kept to a minimum by using only one sheet over the patient (Fig. 4–3). A weight change of 1 kg (2.2 lb) represents a fluid loss or gain of 1 liter. The weight is the best indication of fluid retention, since edema is not generally evident until there is a 10 percent increase in weight. In a normal man of 70 kg, this would be a 7-kg increase or 15.5 lb. Measurement of body weight should be corrected for tissue losses in catabolic states since most postoperative patients lose 0.3 kg a day. A weight gain should be evaluated carefully when it is caused by a "third space" developing from translocations of extracellular fluid, since the water and electrolytes in the third space are not available to the circulation.

Measurement of Circumference of Extremities

This is another method of determining translocations of extracellular fluid. A 1-in. increase in the circumference of one thigh can represent extravasation of 1 to 1.5 liters [25].

Central Venous Pressure

This pressure is measured hourly. It is an important guide for fluid replacement. The method of measurement and interpretation of readings are given in a later section.

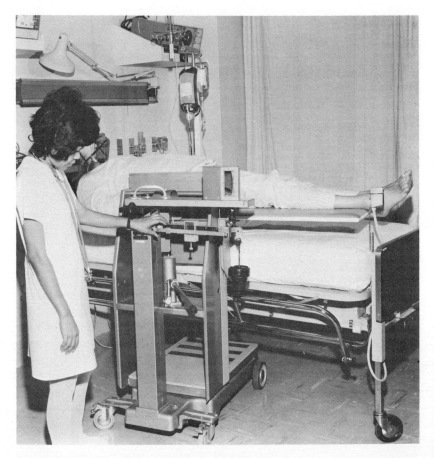

FIGURE 4-3 Use of bed scales for weighing patient.

Physical Appearance

Physical appearance often gives important clues to fluid balance. Observations of fluid volume deficits include:

1 Poor tissue turgor—in the normal patient, pinched skin will fall back to its usual position when released. If fluid volume deficit exists, skin will remain slightly raised for many seconds.

2 Absence of moisture in the groin or axilla is probably indicative of a fluid volume deficit of at least 1500 ml.

3 Dry mucous membranes, which is best determined by feeling the junction between the gums and the buccal mucosa. Patient often complains of "thirst."

4 Sunken eyeballs.

5 Listlessness.

6 Additional furrows on tongue.

7 Tachycardia.

8 Prolonged filling time of peripheral veins—when the hand is elevated, the veins in the hand should empty in 3 to 5 sec and then refill in the same time when the hand is lowered (Fig. 4-4).

Observations of fluid volume excess include:

1 Presence of edema, which pits when pressure is applied. As mentioned previously, edema is not usually evident until there has been a 10 percent increase in weight. Edema may be first noticed at the ankles, but if the patient is on bed rest,

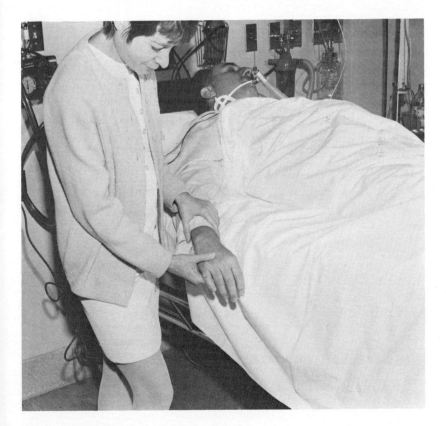

FIGURE 4-4   Testing filling time of peripheral veins.

the sacral area may be the first area to be involved. It may progress to pulmonary edema, causing moist rales, tachycardia, and dyspnea.

2   Puffy eyelids.

3   Venous engorgement with distended jugular veins observable when the patient is in the semi-Fowler's position.

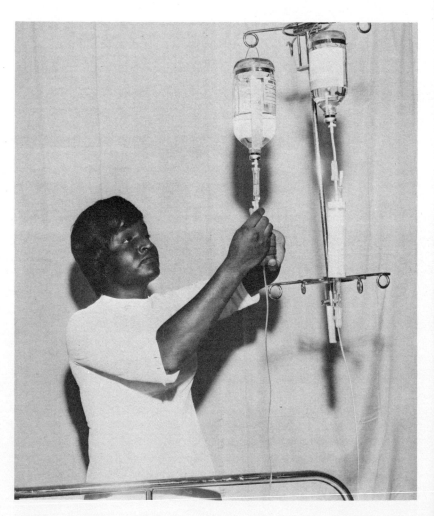

FIGURE 4–5   Accurate rate of infusion is enhanced by the use of the second hand on a watch to count the microdrips, a tape on the bottle with the level marked, and by keeping the clamp immediately below the drip chamber.

Any fluid and electrolyte imbalance may give symptoms of muscle weakness, confusion, and anorexia. Thus these symptoms alone are not enough for diagnosis. Electrolyte studies are usually done every

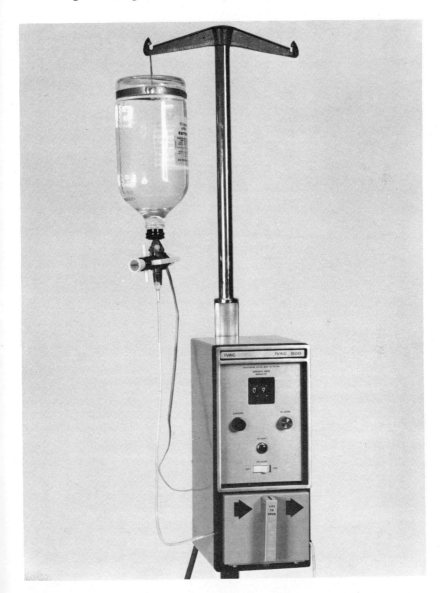

FIGURE 4–6   The Ivac™ 500 Infusion Pump with the drop sensor mounted on the drip chamber of the IV bottle. *(Photograph courtesy of Ivac Corporation, San Diego, Calif.)*

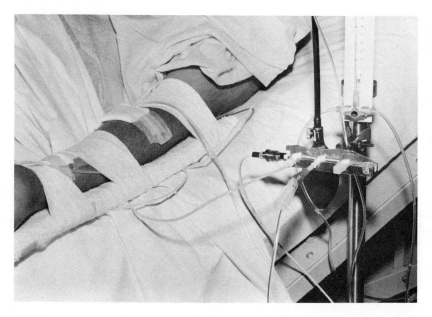

FIGURE 4-7   The use of a padded arm board and stockingette bandage provides both comfort and firm support for intravenous or arterial cannulae.

4 hr for the first 12 hr after surgery, and then every 24 hr. The limitations of serum electrolyte levels have previously been discussed. Electrolyte replacement should take into account electrolyte content of IV antibiotics when patients with renal failure are being treated.

Other laboratory studies of value are BUN, creatinine, hemoglobin, total protein, serum pH, and serial electrocardiograms.

In order for measurements to be meaningful, an effective method of recording them that shows interrelationships and correlations with other physiological measurements is necessary. A sample flow sheet that has proved useful in clinical trail is included in Appendix G.

NURSING MEASURES TO MAINTAIN FLUID AND ELECTROLYTE BALANCE IN THE POSTOPERATIVE PERIOD

Measures	Rationale
Accurately label all intravenous bottles with additives and time of addition. Use a strip of tape on bottle to indicate correct level of fluid at 1- to 2-hr intervals.	Carefully label and time to reduce opportunity for error in administration.

NURSING MEASURES TO MAINTAIN FLUID AND ELECTROLYTE BALANCE IN THE
POSTOPERATIVE PERIOD *(Continued)*

Measures	Rationale
Maintain even rate of intravenous flow. Use a microdrip (sometimes called a minidrip) for solutions to be infused at a slow rate. Keep clamp that regulates the flow immediately below the drip chamber (Fig. 4–5).	Blood-volume maintenance is critical in the open-heart surgery patient so be careful to prevent hypervolemia from too rapid a rate of fluid administration or hypovolemia from too slow a rate. Most microdrops are one-fifth the size of a regular drop, with 50 to 60 drops equaling 1 ml. When a patient has several intravenous lines, the wrong line may be opened inadvertently if the clamps are low.
When potent drugs are being given intravenously and the infusion rate needs to be carefully controlled, use an electronic instrument such as the Ivac$_{TM}$ 500 (Fig. 4–6).	Since the Ivac$_{TM}$ 500 is a transistorized electronic instrument designed to control automatically the rate of infusion without being influenced by temperature changes, venous or arterial pressure, IV tubing, or height of the bottle, it can be depended on to administer drugs accurately.
Identify the type of intravenous infusor (needle, cannula, or cutdown) and date of insertion by writing on the tape that secures it to the patient. Label any arterial line "artery."	Accurate identification ensures greater safety in care and removal of the infusor.
Anchor any intravenous or arterial cannulas firmly at the puncture site (Fig. 4–7).	Mechanical damage to the vessel wall and embolization are minimized when to and fro movement is prevented [26].
Inspect daily the puncture site of needles and cannulas. If there is any evidence of inflammation, remove the cannula or needle, and send the tip of any plastic cannula for culture. Unless the physician desires the site to be exposed to the air, re-dress the site with a sterile dressing containing a small amount of Neosporin cream.	In a study of patients with polyethylene IV cannulas, 39 percent developed phlebitis. The use of antibiotic cream has lessened the incidence of infection [26].
Change all intravenous tubing every 24 to 48 hr and evaluate all indwelling cannulas for change every 48 hr.	Studies of local and systemic infection associated with polyethylene IV cannulas have shown that the risk of local infection increases with the duration of use [26]. Another study showed that all cases of septicemia occurred after cannulas had been in place a minimum of 48 hr, which suggests that there is a necessary incubation period before intravenous extension occurs from a localized septic site [27]. Indwelling subclavian catheters develop fibrin sleeves that can result in occult thrombosis and thromboembolism [28].
Detect infiltration early. Extravasation should especially be guarded against when potassium,	Cellular damage and death can result from extravasation of fluid into the tissues. The use of Regitine in an area of Levophed extravasation helps prevent tissue slough [25].

NURSING MEASURES TO MAINTAIN FLUID AND ELECTROLYTE BALANCE IN THE
POSTOPERATIVE PERIOD (Continued)

Measures	Rationale
Isuprel, or Levophed is being given. Give Regitine subcutaneously into any area of Levophed extravasation.	
Prevent clotting in arterial lines by maintaining a slow drip of heparinized solution and flushing the line after arterial blood samples are drawn.	Accuracy of blood pressure reading depends on patency of the arterial line. A fibrin sleeve may build up on the end of the arterial cannula that may result in occlusion and/or thrombosis.
Check all lines (especially arterial) for tightness of connection.	Accidental separation of tubing results in contamination and, in the case of arterial lines, considerable blood may be lost.
Give support to any edematous area, e.g., scrotal support for edema of scrotum; elastic stocking or ace bandages for edema of the legs.	Support provides comfort for the patient and improves venous return, thereby reducing edema.
Give mouth care to the dehydrated patient or the patient with an oral endotracheal tube.	Proper care helps prevent mucous membrane lesions and secondary infections.
Use lotion and light massage for dry-skin areas and bony prominences.	Light massage improves local blood supply and helps to maintain tissue integrity.
Bathe with soap and water only those body areas that will enhance the comfort of patient.	Soap and water are drying to skin, and may predispose to skin breakdown.
Use gravity to drain urine from tubing for hourly measurements on a Foley catheter. Do not separate tubing from Foley catheters. For collection of urine use a Cystoflow or similar drainage bag that has a built-in trap to prevent urine backflow and a bottom drain for emptying.	Maintenance of a closed system that has a trap to prevent backflow for urinary drainage reduces the incidence of infection. Although some urine remains in the tubing when the tubing is not separated, the measurements only vary 5 ml, which is not of sufficient significance to risk infection—especially since the total over a period of time is the same.
Limit fluid intake and sodium when patient is started on oral feedings.	Fluid and sodium restriction is necessary to prevent fluid overload on the fourth or fifth postoperative day as the perfusate leaves the interstitial compartment and reenters the intravascular compartment [11].

THE RESPIRATORY SYSTEM

5

Respiration is a series of processes whereby oxygen is transferred from the atmosphere through the respiratory passages to the alveoli of the lung; oxygen diffuses across the alveolar membrane into the blood stream in exchange for carbon dioxide; and carbon dioxide is eliminated through the lungs and respiratory passages.

Respiratory function depends upon the circulatory system for transport of oxygen through the blood to the tissue cells where it is utilized and the transport of carbon dioxide produced by cellular respiration (sometimes referred to as internal respiration) to the lungs.

PHYSIOLOGY

The respiratory system has two main divisions: (1) *the conducting airway*, which is composed of the mouth, nasal passages, pharynx, larynx, trachea, bronchi, and bronchioles. The airway serves to warm, humidify, and filter the air, but there is no exchange of oxygen and carbon dioxide. Thus the internal volume of the conducting airway (approximately 150cc in the average adult male) is referred to as the anatomic dead space.

(2) *the alveoli,* where gas exchange occurs. The two lungs contain about 300 million alveoli; these alveoli have a membrane surface of over 90 square meters [29].

RESPIRATION PROCESSES

Ventilation

Ventilation is the movement of air in and out of the lungs for the maintenance of high oxygen and low carbon dioxide pressures necessary for diffusion. By the use of a spirometer, the normal amounts of air present within the respiratory system and the rate at which it is exchanged during the respiratory cycle of inspiration have been measured (Fig. 5-1).

The tidal volume is the amount of air inspired and expired during each respiratory cycle. It is normally about 400 ml.

The inspiratory reserve volume is the maximal amount of air that can be inspired from the end of the normal inspiratory period. It is normally about 3200 ml.

The inspiratory capacity is the sum of the tidal volume and inspiratory reserve volume with the volume of air that can be inspired with a maximum effort averaging 3600 ml.

The expiratory reserve volume is the amount of air that can be expired with a maximum effort at the end of the normal expiratory period. It is normally about 1200 ml.

The residual volume is the amount of air remaining in the lungs at the end of a maximal expiration. Since the lungs do not collapse to an airless state at the end of each respiration, 1200 ml normally remain even after the most forceful effort possible.

FIGURE 5-1   LUNG VOLUMES   Above: the large central diagram illustrates the four primary lung volumes and approximate magnitude. The outermost line indicates the greatest size to which the lung can expand; the innermost circle (residual volume), the volume that remains after all air has been voluntarily squeezed out of the lungs. Surrounding the central diagram are smaller ones; shaded areas in these represent the four lung capacities. The volume of dead space gas is included in residual volume, functional residual capacity and total lung capacity when these are measured by routine techniques. Below: lung volumes as they appear on a spirographic tracing; shading in vertical bar next to tracing corresponds to that in central diagram above. (*Diagrams and legend from Julius H. Comroe, Jr., et al., "The Lung," Year Book Medical Publishers, Inc., Chicago, 1968. Used by permission.*)

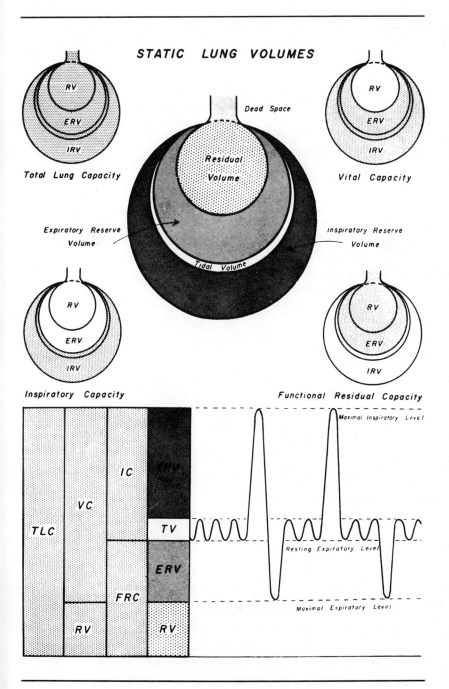

STATIC LUNG VOLUMES

The functional residual capacity is the amount of air remaining after a normal respiration and is the sum of the residual volume and the expiratory reserve volume. Thus, 2400 ml of air remain in the alveolar compartment after exhaling. Since the tidal volume is normally 400 ml, 400 ml of fresh air is inhaled and added to the 2400 ml of air remaining in the lungs. This makes a ratio of one part of fresh air to six parts of used air. This provides a buffer against extreme fluctuations in the oxygen tension through the respiratory cycle.

Since the vital process of gaseous exchange takes place in the alveoli, the most meaningful measurement is that of *alveolar ventilation,* which is the volume of fresh air entering the alveoli with each breath. It is affected by dead space volume, tidal volume, and respiratory rate. Before inspiration, the conducting airway or dead space is filled with air that has the same ratio of used air to fresh air as that in the alveolar compartment (6:1). On inspiration, 400 ml of fresh air will enter from the atmosphere. The first 150 ml that reaches the alveoli will be the mixture from the dead space with 250 ml of fresh air following. The remaining 150 ml of fresh air will remain in the dead space and will be the first air expired.

The respiratory rate affects the ventilation since rapid respiration is shallower, with a corresponding lower tidal volume. Thus ventilation is measured by the amount inspired and expired for a minute.

Minute ventilation vol. $\quad$ = tidal vol. $\times$ respiratory rate
Minute alveolar ventilation vol. = tidal vol. − dead space vol.
$$\times \text{ respiratory rate}$$

Thus if the tidal volume is 400 ml, dead space is 150 ml, and respiratory rate is 16, the minute ventilation would be

400 ml $\times$ 16 $\quad$ or $\quad$ 6,400 ml min (6.4 liters)

The minute alveolar ventilation would be

400 ml − 150 ml $\times$ 16 $\quad$ or $\quad$ 4,000 ml or 4 liters/min

If room air that contains approximately 20 percent oxygen is breathed, 800 ml of oxygen is delivered to the alveoli every minute ($1/5$ of 4000 ml = 800 ml). However, if the minute volume remains the same but the rate of respiration increases, the minute alveolar ventilation is greatly reduced. Tidal volume would be 228 at

28 resp/min (228 ml − 150 ml × 28 = 2184 ml), which delivers 437 liters of oxygen/min to the alveoli. Thus it is evident that rapid shallow respirations primarily "ventilate the dead space" and do not adequately ventilate the alveoli.

The normal man at rest needs 200 to 250 ml of O_2/ min, but with exercise 20 times this amount is needed. Increase in the respiratory rate during periods of exercise results in a greater volume of oxygen inspired and carbon dioxide expired, which is a homeostatic method for maintaining the concentration gradient across the alveolar membrane.

Diffusion

Diffusion is the passive transfer of gas across the alveolar membrane from an area of higher concentration to an area of lower concentration. The alveolar membrane is the interface between the molecules in a gaseous state and those in a liquid state. However, for oxygen to pass from the alveoli into the pulmonary capillaries of the blood, the concentration of oxygen in the alveoli must be higher than in the venous blood of the capillaries. Likewise, the concentration of carbon dioxide in the alveoli must be lower than in the venous blood for it to diffuse across the alveolar membrane and be exhaled.

The constant bombardment of a mixture of gas molecules against the wall of a container exerts a pressure on the wall of the container. The concentration of one gas in a mixture of gases is termed the *tension* or *partial pressure* of that gas, since the pressure in the container that is exhibited by the gas is only part of the total pressure in the container. The partial pressure of oxygen is expressed as PO_2, and the partial pressure of carbon dioxide is termed PCO_2. According to Dalton's law, the sum of the partial pressures of the gases in the atmosphere is equal to the total atmospheric pressure. Atmospheric pressure at sea level and at standard temperature is 760 mm Hg. However, the total pressure of the gases in the moist trachea or alveoli is 713 mm Hg, since inspired air is humidified in the upper airways and the water-vapor pressure at body temperature is 47 mm Hg. The water-vapor pressure and the pressure of the gases together constitute the atmospheric pressure.

The main gases in the atmosphere are nitrogen (79 percent) and oxygen (20.93 percent). There are extremely small amounts of argon, hydrogen, and carbon dioxide. Since nitrogen is chemically inert, it will not be considered in detail. The partial pressure of oxygen in the trachea would be

20.93% of 713 = 149 mm Hg

The alveolar oxygen tension is still lower as a result of the mixture of fresh air and used air that results in a higher percentage of carbon dioxide with a lower percentage of oxygen in the alveoli (partial pressure of carbon dioxide in the atmosphere and the trachea is only 0.3 percent). The partial pressure of oxygen in the alveolar air in a normal patient under ideal conditions would be

PO_2 = 14.6% of 713 = 104 mm Hg

The partial pressure of carbon dioxide in the alveolar air in the normal patient would be

PCO_2 = 5.6% of 713 = 40 mm Hg

Since mixed venous blood in the pulmonary capillaries has a partial oxygen pressure of 40 and a partial carbon dioxide pressure of 46, diffusion can take place across the alveolar membrane.[1]

REGULATION OF RESPIRATION (Fig. 5-2)

Neural Control

The *central neural regulator of respiration* is located in the medulla. This respiratory center activates the phrenic and intercostal nerves, which in turn regulate the rate and force of contraction of the respiratory muscles. Impulses reach the medulla from many areas; these areas include:

1 *Peripheral chemosensitive* receptors in the aorta and the carotid bodies, which respond to a decrease in arterial PO_2.

2 *Arterial and venous baroreceptors* in the aorta and carotid bodies, which respond to a decrease in blood pressure by stimulating the respiratory center.

3 *Pulmonary stretch receptors* that send impulses to the medulla

[1]All figures for partial pressures are taken from Julius H. Comroe, "Physiology of Respiration," Year Book Medical Publishers, Inc., Chicago, 1965.

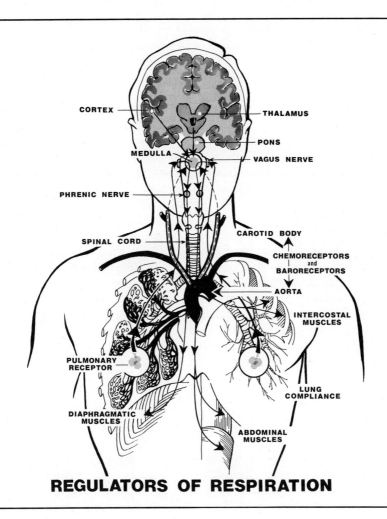

CORTEX — THALAMUS

MEDULLA — PONS

VAGUS NERVE

PHRENIC NERVE

SPINAL CORD — CAROTID BODY

CHEMORECEPTORS
and
BARORECEPTORS

AORTA

INTERCOSTAL
MUSCLES

PULMONARY
RECEPTOR

LUNG
COMPLIANCE

DIAPHRAGMATIC
MUSCLES

ABDOMINAL
MUSCLES

REGULATORS OF RESPIRATION

FIGURE 5–2

and pons via the vagus nerves to terminate inspiration and otherwise assist in the regulation of breathing.

4   *Cortical impulses* for conscious hyperventilation.

5   *Thalamic impulses* for alteration of the respiratory rate in response to emotions.

6   *Central chemoreceptors* located near the surface of the medulla that are sensitive to CO_2 and the hydrogen-ion concentration.

They do not respond as rapidly as the peripheral receptors to abrupt changes in the PCO_2 of arterial blood. They are influenced more by the composition of the cerebrospinal fluid (CSF) than by that of blood. The PCO_2 of blood and CSF are approximately the same. However, since CSF does not have a hemoglobin buffer to accept hydrogen ions, when the PCO_2 increases, the hydrogen ion of the CSF rises more than that of blood. When arterial PCO_2 is lowered by prolonged hyperventilation, the hydrogen ion of the CSF will decrease more than that of blood. Thus, after any changes in arterial PCO_2, time is required for equalization of the gas tensions between the blood and the CSF. Patients who have been hyperventilated on respirators for many days continue to hyperventilate when they are taken off the respirator. One explanation given by Comroe [30] is that the level of the hydrogen ion in the CSF falls below that of the blood while the patient is being hyperventilated on the respirator. When he is taken off the respirator his PCO_2 increases, and the resultant increase in the hydrogen-ion concentration of the CSF will stimulate the central chemoreceptors, causing the patient to continue to hyperventilate for a few hours or perhaps a day until the hydrogen-ion concentration is equalized.

Other Regulatory Mechanisms

The action of the diaphragm and the external intercostal muscles increases the size of the thorax with inspiration. The normal lung tends to recoil from the chest wall, creating a subatmospheric pressure (sometimes incorrectly termed *negative* pressure) within the pleural cavity of 5 mm Hg less than atmospheric pressure at the end of expiration. When the thorax enlarges with inspiration, the intrathoracic pressure decreases (usually to 10 to 15 mm Hg lower than atmospheric pressure), exerting a pulling pressure sufficient to overcome the normal frictional resistance that impedes the flow of air into the lungs.

The elasticity of the lungs also offers resistance to the flow of air into the lungs. Compliance is the term that expresses the relationship between changes in volume as a result of changes in pressure. Collagen and elastic tissue, vascular structures, and surfactant (a surface-active material that lines the alveoli) make up the elastic resistance of the lung. The pressure required to stretch elastic tissue during inspiration is stored as potential energy. Normal expiration is passive, utilizing the stored energy. When an obstructive condition of the airway exists, the stored potential energy is inadequate and additional active expiratory pressure is required to exhale the CO_2 [29]. Other causes of reduced elasticity and increased airway resistance will be discussed in the section dealing with respiratory problems.

TRANSPORT OF OXYGEN AND CARBON DIOXIDE BY THE BLOOD

Some of the oxygen that passes from the alveoli into the blood and some of the carbon dioxide that enters the blood from the tissues is dissolved in the plasma. However, the plasma could never carry enough oxygen to sustain the metabolic activity of the cells, as 100 ml of plasma will bind only 0.3 ml of O_2 at a PO_2 of 100 mm Hg. Hemoglobin, a protein in the red blood cells, performs the important function of forming a reversible combination with either oxygen or carbon dioxide, depending on their concentrations in the blood. The hemoglobin molecule contains four iron-heme units, each of which contains an atom of iron combined with a molecule of globin. The iron combines with a molecule of oxygen to form oxyhemoglobin, which is carried to the tissues where it becomes dissociated.

Oxygen capacity is the maximal amount of oxygen that will combine with hemoglobin when the hemoglobin is fully saturated with oxygen. Since each gram of hemoglobin that is fully saturated binds 1.34 ml of oxygen in each 100 ml of blood, a person with 15 gm of hemoglobin per 100 ml of blood could carry 15×1.34 ml or 20.1 ml of oxygen in each 100 ml of blood. This capacity changes to reflect varying concentrations of hemoglobin, so percent of oxygen saturation is used as a more reliable guide for the expression of the amount of oxygen combined with hemoglobin.

Oxygen saturation percent is determined by

$$\frac{\text{Amount of } O_2 \text{ combined with hemoglobin}}{O_2 \text{ capacity of hemoglobin}} \times 100$$

The amount of oxygen combined with hemoglobin is determined by the partial pressure of oxygen in the red blood cell. When alveolar oxygen tension is 100 mm Hg, approximately 19.5 ml of oxygen can be combined with each 100 ml of blood.[1] Thus for a normal person with a hemoglobin of 15 gm,

$$O_2 \text{ saturation} = \frac{19.5}{20.1} \times 100 = 97.5\%$$

The relationship between oxygen saturation and PO_2 has been plotted on a graph and termed the *oxyhemoglobin dissociation curve*. Some relationships demonstrated by the curve are (Fig. 5–3):

When PO_2 increases above 100, the hemoglobin is unable to accept much more oxygen, since it is 97.5 percent saturated at a PO_2 of 100. It is probably fully saturated when the PO_2 is 250 mm Hg. Thus hyperventilation cannot add more than 2.5 percent to the oxygen saturation in a normal person.

The sigmoid shape of the curve with the flat upper portion indicates that there is a very little change in the amount of oxygen held by the hemoglobin between O_2 tensions of 100 and 70 mm Hg. A patient with a PO_2 of 70 mm Hg has an oxygen saturation of 92.7 percent—a decrease of only 5 percent. This ensures an adequate supply of oxygen to the tissues even though the patient may have a drop in PO_2.

At a low PO_2 between 10 and 40 mm Hg, such as is found in the tissues, the curve is very steep. This allows the oxyhemoglobin to dissociate and give up its oxygen, with large amounts of oxygen released for relatively small decreases in PO_2. Blood with a PO_2 of 40 mm Hg can bind 75 percent of its oxygen. Blood with a PO_2 of 10 can bind only 13 percent of its oxygen.

The oxyhemoglobin dissociation curve is not fixed. A decreasing pH, which occurs with an increase of CO_2, shifts the curve to the right so that less oxygen is bound at the same oxygen tension. The amount of oxygen loading at the pulmonary capillaries is not greatly decreased, but more oxygen is unloaded at the tissues than with a normal pH. The effect of a decreasing pH on the oxyhemoglobin dissociation curve is known as the Bohr effect. Alkalosis shifts the curve to the left,

[1]The amount of O_2 combined with hemoglobin at each PO_2 was calculated by Comroe by placing whole blood in flasks with varying oxygen tensions and swirling the flasks until they took up as much oxygen as they could. The amount of oxygen was then measured and expressed as ml $O_2/100$ ml blood. The amount of oxygen dissolved in the plasma was calculated for each PO_2 and subtracted from the total $O_2/100$ ml blood to give the amount of oxygen combined with hemoglobin.

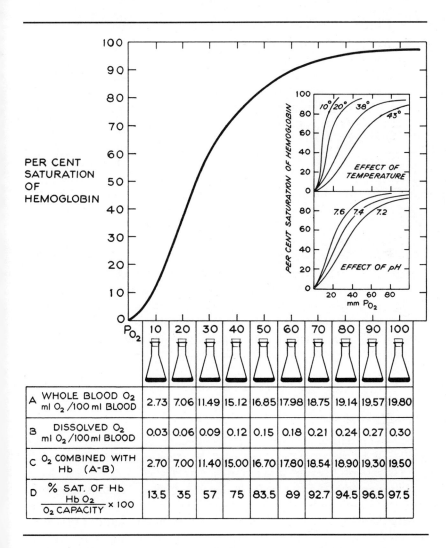

	PO₂	10	20	30	40	50	60	70	80	90	100
A	WHOLE BLOOD O₂ ml O₂/100 ml BLOOD	2.73	7.06	11.49	15.12	16.85	17.98	18.75	19.14	19.57	19.80
B	DISSOLVED O₂ ml O₂/100 ml BLOOD	0.03	0.06	0.09	0.12	0.15	0.18	0.21	0.24	0.27	0.30
C	O₂ COMBINED WITH Hb (A−B)	2.70	7.00	11.40	15.00	16.70	17.80	18.54	18.90	19.30	19.50
D	% SAT. OF Hb $\frac{Hb\ O_2}{O_2\ CAPACITY} \times 100$	13.5	35	57	75	83.5	89	92.7	94.5	96.5	97.5

FIGURE 5–3 OXYHEMOGLOBIN DISSOCIATION CURVE   The large graph shows a single dissociation curve, applicable when the pH of the blood is 7.40 and temperature 38° C. The blood O₂ tension and saturation of patients with CO₂ retention, acidosis, alkalosis, fever or hypothermia will not fit this curve because the curve shifts to the right or left when temperature, pH or PCO₂ is changed. Effects on the HbO₂ dissociation curve of change in temperature (upper right) and in pH (lower right) are shown in the smaller graphs. A small change in blood pH occurs regularly in the body; e.g., when mixed venous blood passes through the pulmonary capillaries, PCO₂ decreases from 46 to 40 mm Hg and pH rises from 7.37 to 7.40. During this time, blood changes from a pH of 7.37 dissociation curve to a pH of 7.40 curve. (*Diagram and legend from Julius H. Comroe, Jr., "Physiology of Respiration," Year Book Medical Publishers, Inc., Chicago, 1965. Used by permission.*)

so more oxygen is bound at the same oxygen tension. The curve is also affected by temperature, with high temperatures having an effect similar to low pH. When an increase in the metabolic rate that increases the oxygen requirements of the tissues is accompanied by a higher temperature and an increase in PCO_2 (which decreases the pH), a homeostatic mechanism is at work to increase oxyhemoglobin dissociation and supply the oxygen needed by the tissues.

A *carbon dioxide dissociation curve*, which demonstrates the relationship between the carbon dioxide content of the blood and the PCO_2 can also be plotted. The relationships between the two are almost linear, in contrast with the sigmoid shape of the oxyhemoglobin dissociation curve. Thus when ventilation is inadequate and alveolar PCO_2 rises, the tissue and venous CO_2 will correspondingly rise. Conversely, hyperventilation with a decrease in PCO_2 results in a lowered tissue and venous CO_2. The oxygen saturation of the blood influences the CO_2 content. Haldane was the first to demonstrate that reduced hemoglobin can carry significantly more carbon dioxide than oxygenated hemoglobin at the same PCO_2. Combined O_2 and CO_2 curves are helpful because they depict the oxygen saturation at any given PO_2 and PCO_2.

VENTILATION PROBLEMS

Alveolar Hyperventilation (Respiratory Alkalosis)

This is ventilation in excess of that needed to eliminate the CO_2 produced by the metabolic process. As excessive amounts of CO_2 are "blown off," hypocapnia results. (A PCO_2 below 35 mm Hg is usually considered to be a CO_2 deficit.) This is accompanied by a corresponding decrease in hydrogen ions and carbonic acid concentration (pH is increased above 7.45). A homeostatic mechanism for restoration of the normal acid-base balance is the action of the kidneys in excreting bicarbonate ions while retaining hydrogen and nonbicarbonate ions such as chloride. With increased secretion of bicarbonate, the urine becomes more alkaline (pH above the normal level of 6), which helps to distinguish respiratory alkalosis from metabolic alkalosis, as the high excretion of potassium ions in metabolic alkalosis may result in an acid urine.

Hyperventilation that results in a PCO_2 below 35 mm Hg should be avoided since cerebral vasoconstriction results, with a decrease in cerebral blood flow. High tidal volumes have also been found to destroy the pulmonary surfactant essential for the maintenance of surface tension in the alveoli.

The major causes of hyperventilation in the open-heart surgery patient are: overventilation by a mechanical respirator; anxiety and apprehension; fever and infection; homeostatic mechanisms in response to hypoxemia (low oxygen tension stimulates respiratory center) and metabolic acidosis (decreased pH stimulates respiratory center); and hepatic failure.

Alveolar Hypoventilation (Respiratory Acidosis)

This is an impairment of ventilation in which an inadequate gas exchange in the alveoli results in carbon dioxide retention with a corresponding increase in hydrogen-ion and carbonic acid concentration (pH below 7.35). Hypercapnia is usually considered present when the PCO_2 is higher than 45 mm Hg. Compensatory mechanisms instituted by the kidney to conserve base bicarbonate are not as efficient as those of excretion of bicarbonate with respiratory alkalosis. An increasing carbon dioxide tension tends to have an anesthetic effect on ventilation, so the high level of CO_2 is no longer an effective stimulus for ventilation (CO_2 narcosis). The effects of hypercapnia are:

1   Dilatation of the cerebral blood vessels.
2   Increased cerebral blood flow.
3   Increased spinal fluid pressure.
4   Muscular twitchings and convulsions, which may lead to unconsciousness.
5   Increased pulmonary vascular resistance in the lungs, which results in a high pulmonary artery pressure and increased stress in the right side of the heart. This in turn may lead to cor pulmonale.

Hypercapnia is usually but not always accompanied by hypoxemia, which is characterized by a PO_2 below 74 mm Hg. Most people do not have important physiological changes until the PO_2 falls below 60 mm Hg. The main idicators of hypoxemia are:

1   Tachycardia.
2   Tachypnea.

3 Hyperpnea.

4 Irritability and nervousness—a sudden change in personality with an increasing irritability should "clue" the nurse in to the possibility of hypoxemia.

5 Loss of judgment, dizziness, nausea, and extreme restlessness are later symptoms that develop when previously normal PO_2 drops to 50 mm Hg or below.

6 Increased myocardial irritability with abnormal heart rhythms.

Respiratory Insufficiency

Respiratory insufficiency in the open-heart surgery patient can result from many factors (see Table 5–1). They all result in pulmonary capillary damage with transudation of fluid and atelectasis. When alveoli are completely collapsed, the blood that perfuses them does not become oxygenated. This disorder of relationship between ventilation and perfusion has been termed physiologic arteriovenous shunting or a right-to-left shunt. Shunting produces hypoxemia without hypercapnia. Failure of the PO_2 to rise to at least 580 mm Hg when tested by breathing 100 percent oxygen is an indication of shunting [5]. Peripheral perfusion and oxygenation are impaired by shunting and its accompanying hypoxemia. If compensation is not effected, the decrease in the perfusion-metabolism ratio, with cellular breakdown products toxic to the pulmonary capillaries, further complicates the situation. The net result is pulmonary edema, increased pulmonary venous and left atrial pressure, and left ventricular failure.

When the condition of acute respiratory distress follows a period of shock, it has been termed shock lung or "pump lung." The cardiopulmonary bypass procedure is a form of controlled clinical shock. Most patients recover rather quickly, but a few patients have progressive hypoxemia with a right-to-left shunt, reduction in pulmonary compliance, low lung volume, and impairment of CO_2 elimination. The symptoms progress for 36 to 48 hr and then may gradually resolve if the patient survives. The etiology of the syndrome is unknown, but various contributing factors have been identified, including disseminated intravascular clotting (DIC), vasospasm, fat embolus, protein denaturation, oxygen toxicity, serotonin release, heart failure, low osmolality of the blood, homologous blood reactions, and toxic shock.

The causes of pulmonary insufficiency are described in Table 5–1.

TABLE 5-1   CAUSES OF PULMONARY INSUFFICIENCY FOLLOWING OPEN-HEART SURGERY

Cause	Physiological Alteration
Preexisting pulmonary disease	No further reduction can be tolerated in the elasticity of tissues, in the permeability of the membrane, or in the functional residual capacity.
Effect of anesthesia and narcotics	Central nervous system is depressed, with subsequent loss of spontaneous intermittent deep breaths (sighs).
Cardiopulmonary bypass	Direct blood-gas interface in the oxygenator and the coronary suction return results in denaturization of the blood's elements, with hemolyzed blood deposited interstitially in the lungs. Gas embolism may occur with the bypass procedure.
Failure of the left ventricle to maintain output provided by pump following release of the aortic clamp	Distension of the left atrium that results from left ventricular failure and sudden increase in the pulmonary vascular pressure damage the pulmonary capillaries.
Muscle and nerve destruction by surgery	Ability to increase size of the thorax with inspiration is limited and resultant pain leads to splinting and shallow breathing.
Unreplaced blood loss	Oxygen-carrying power of the blood is reduced by the dilution and lowered hemoglobin of the blood.
Retained secretions	Inadequate gas exchange in the alveoli results in unoxygenated blood being returned to the heart. When secretions occlude the bronchi, air below the occlusion is forced into the blood stream, resulting in collapse of the alveoli.
Increased fluid in the alveoli of the lungs	Destruction of the air-membrane interface, with transudation of fluid into the lungs, results when more fluid enters the lungs than can be drained by the lymphatics. Intravenous infusion of large amounts of non-colloid fluid dilutes the plasma proteins, decreasing the osmotic pressure and overloading the extracellular space of the lung. When the left atrial pressure exceeds 25 mm Hg, the increased hydrostatic pressure results in pulmonary capillary transudation [5].
Multiple transfusions of stored blood	Blood stored for several days contains particles and cellular agglomerates that require a higher pressure for filtration [31]. When these particles are broken down in the lung capillary bed, vasoactive materials are released, which may lead to capillary damage.
Alveolar collapse secondary to destruction or inactivation of pulmonary surfactant	Surfactant is a complex lipoprotein secreted by the alveoli, which changes its surface tension with changes in the alveolar dimensions. As the size of the alveoli decreases with expiration, the surface tension decreases, preventing the alveolar walls from collapsing completely and their sides sticking together so that they could not reopen. When surfactant is decreased, resistance to air flow is increased and more subatmospheric pressure than is usually present is required to overcome the tendency to collapse. Factors that decrease surfactant are prolonged inhalation of 100 percent oxygen, reduced humidity, subnormal body temperature, too large or too small tidal volume, and plasma proteins leaking into the alveolar space that react with surfactant to form proteinaceous deposits [32].

TABLE 5-1   CAUSES OF PULMONARY INSUFFICIENCY FOLLOWING OPEN-HEART SURGERY
(Continued)

Cause	Physiological Alteration
Decrease in cardiac output	Decrease in the ratio of perfusion to alveolar ventilation results in insufficient blood delivery to the lungs. Decrease in the ratio of perfusion to metabolism results in anaerobic metabolism with cellular breakdown. The products of cellular metabolism appear to be directly toxic to the pulmonary capillary endothelium [33].
Effect of alpha-adrenergic stimulating drugs as Aramine or Levophed	Maintenance of central blood pressure at the expense of adequate peripheral perfusion also results in anaerobic metabolism with release of autolytic enzymes. When adequate flow is reestablished, the products of anaerobic metabolism, cellular breakdown, and intravascular coagulation are flushed back into the venous circulation, with the lungs acting as a sieve for the particulate material that is washed out [34].
Bronchospasm	The ventilation-perfusion balance is interfered with as a result of an allergic reaction or the effect of beta-adrenergic blocking drugs such as propanolol (Inderal).
Lung infection	Diffusion of gases in the lungs is reduced by collected mucus. Active pneumonitis in the areas of "boggy" atelectasis leads to destruction of pulmonary tissue, which is irreversible [5].
Aspiration of stomach contents	The acidity of the aspirate is so irritating that it sets up an acute inflammatory reaction that prevents adequate gaseous exchange.
Gastric dilatation	Pressure against the diaphragm decreases the expansion area of the lungs.
Fat, fibrin, or platelet emboli	Pulmonary endothelium is damaged from loss of blood supply and from products resulting from subsequent lysis.
Prolonged supine position without intermittent hyperinflation	Tidal breathing without spontaneous deep respirations results in a progressive collapse of the alveoli, a decrease in compliance, and a decrease in functional residual capacity [35].
Hemothorax	Compression of the lung results when blood is retained in the thoracic cavity, as occurs when the chest tube becomes plugged with a blood clot or otherwise fails to function.
Pneumothorax	Pressures generated by mechanical ventilation may cause rupture of a bronchus or an alveolus. Rupture of an alveolus allows air to escape into tissue which can cause dissection along the tracheobronchial tree to the mediastinum, with collapse of the lung.

NURSING ASSESSMENT OF RESPIRATION

Blood Gas Studies

To obtain a reliable assessment of the adequacy of respiration, studies of tensions of the blood gases are needed. A wide range of values are accepted as normal. The values considered normal by Dr. Stemmer [36] are:

PO_2 = 74–104 mm Hg
PCO_2 = 35–45 mm Hg
pH = 7.36–7.44
O_2 saturation = 97.5%

The PO_2 is a measure of oxygenation. It gives information about the lung parenchyma and the combined relationships of ventilation, diffusion, and perfusion. The PCO_2 is a measure of the adequacy of the ventilation volume.

The pH measures the hydrogen-ion concentration in the circulating blood as related to the blood buffers. It is an indication of hypoventilation (acidosis) or hyperventilation (alkalosis) but is also affected by metabolism and various compensatory mechanisms to maintain homeostasis, so it alone is not a reliable indicator of the adequacy of respiration.

The percent of O_2 saturation is an index of the amount of oxygen combined with hemoglobin. A low PO_2 of 70 can usually be tolerated as long as the percent of oxygen saturation does not drop below 90. Hypovolemia may result in a higher percent of oxygen saturation than would be expected for the PO_2. pH affects the oxygen saturation of hemoglobin since with acidosis and a decreasing pH, the hemoglobin becomes less saturated.

The blood gas values should be correlated with the symptoms of hypercapnia and hypoxemia enumerated above. Preoperative tensions are important guides for the oxygen needs during the post-operative period. Although the PO_2 can be maintained at a high level when the patient is on a respirator, it is usually kept below 150 mm Hg in order to avoid the toxic effects of oxygen on the pulmonary membranes; concentrations of oxygen greater than 60 percent maintained for 24 to 72 hours can cause interstitial edema, hemorrhages, fibrosis, and decreased compliance [37]. However, a few patients exhibit dangerous arrhythmias with PO_2 values of 150 mm Hg that disappear when the PO_2 is increased. Thus the PO_2 may occasionally need to be maintained at 250 mm Hg [38].

It is important to evaluate the PCO_2, pH, and O_2 saturation as well as the PO_2. The relationship between the values is important and furnishes a guide of the patient's response to his treatment. The interrelationships will be discussed further in the section on management of patient on respirators.

Blood gas studies are usually done on arterial blood from an arterial catheter or from direct puncture of an artery (Fig. 5–4).

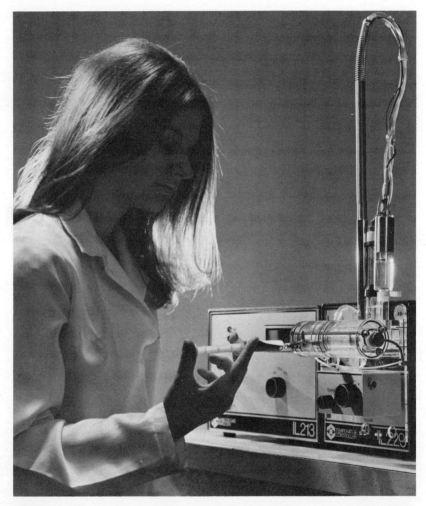

FIGURE 5–4A   Use of a blood gas analyzer machine with arterial blood sample. (A) shows injection of the arterial blood through a port in the water bath that contains the temperature controller and the PO_2 and PCO_2 electrodes. The pH and reference electrode is above and behind the water bath. (B) shows the digital readout figures. *(Photographs courtesy of Instrumentation Laboratory, Inc., Lexington, Mass.)*

Guidelines for obtaining the blood sample are in Appendix C. A new method of measuring PCO_2 that does not require cannulation of an artery has been developed at Johns Hopkins University [39]. It utilizes a Severinghaus electrode with a sensitive membrane (which is permeable to CO_2) placed in contact with the skin of the

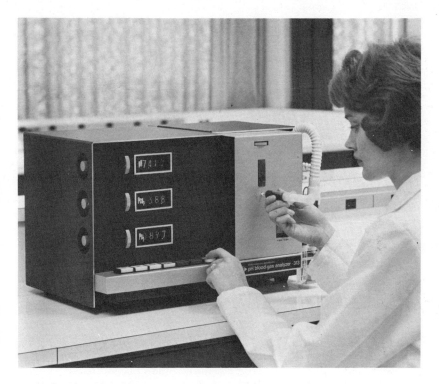

FIGURE 5-4B

forearm and secured with a strap around the arm. Also available
are rapid response oxygen analyzers that can make breath-by-
breath oxygen consumption measurements, but the present
machines are cumbersome and overly complex.

Pulmonary Function Studies

These studies, done in the preoperative period, give an indication of any preexisting lung pathology and help to determine
the feasibility of the surgery and the anticipated assistance to
respiration that will be needed. Postoperative measurements of
minute alveolar volume can be made with a respirometer when
there is a cuffed endotracheal tube or tracheostomy tube in place
(see charts at end of chapter). They are not so accurate when a
face mask or a mouthpiece with a nose clip are used. Nomograms are available to compare the patient's minute alveolar
ventilation with the normal for a person of his height and weight.

In general, tidal volumes 20 percent higher than the normal are needed by most patients in the early postoperative period. Some surgeons recommend tidal volumes of 15 ml per kg [5].

Roentgen examinations of the chest will reveal:

Atelectasis caused by an obstruction of a main bronchus, although early diffuse atelectasis may not be apparent.

Displacement of the endotracheal tube into either the right or left main bronchus.

Hemothorax when it is severe enough to compress the lung and cause a mediastinal shift.

Pulmonary edema, which demonstrates a progressive involvement related to the severity of the condition. Early pulmonary edema is evidenced by hilar density, and a hazy ground-glass picture appears with more advanced edema.

Nursing Observation of Respiration

Relationship between the Inspiratory and Expiratory Periods

This ratio is normally 1:2. In order to have adequate venous return, the ratio needs to be maintained whether patients are on or off the respirator. With rapid respirations that cannot be adequately slowed, the ratio may drop to 1:1. This can be tolerated in a patient with no underlying lung condition but will result in hypercapnia in a patient with an obstructive lung condition.

Rate of Respiration

For adults the rate is normally 12 to 18 per minute. *Tachypnea* refers to a fast rate. It may be accompanied by shallow respirations that only ventilate the dead space. *Bradypnea* refers to a slow rate and may be the result of CO_2 narcosis.

Character of Respiration

Respiration may be regular or irregular. *Hyperpnea* refers to deep respirations. *Dyspnea* is a subjective symptom of difficulty in breathing. One cause of dyspnea is that hyperpnea and tachypnea cause respiratory muscles to use up their supply of oxygen and become fatigued. Metabolites such as lactic acid then accumulate in the cell, giving an uncomfortable feeling.

Retraction occurs when breathing is difficult and the accessory muscles of respiration are used (can be noted in the supraclavicular notch, intercostal spaces, and in the epigastric area).

Excursions of the chest may be decreased or uneven when the lung is being inadequately ventilated. Listening to the chest with a stethoscope helps to identify inadequacies, but as previously mentioned, diffuse atelectasis can be present with essentially normal breath sounds since the airway may be unobstructed to the level of the alveolar duct.

Presence of Cyanosis

Cyanosis of the lips or nailbeds, which is a somewhat inaccurate index of inadequate oxygenation of the blood, should be noted. If the hemoglobin is below 7, hypoxemia is accompanied by pallor rather than a blue color. Patients in vasoconstrictive shock have little blood in their surface vessels, and thus hypoxemia may be present without visible cyanosis. Under most circumstances, cyanosis is not discernible until the oxygen saturation has dropped to 80 percent, the usual saturation when the PO_2 is 48 mm Hg. Thus cyanosis is not a reliable indicator of early hypoxemia.

Abnormal Sounds

Abnormal sounds may indicate a respiratory problem. The main sounds are *rales*, which are rattling, moist, bubbling sounds heard mainly on inspiration and usually indicate fluid in the lungs. Interstitial edema may be present without rales, however; *laryngeal stridor*, which is a high-pitched, coarse noise that indicates upper airway obstruction when it is accompanied by retraction; and *wheezing*, which results from air being forced through narrow ducts. It is usually caused by an obstructive condition of the lungs.

MECHANICAL VENTILATION

Indications for the Use of Respirators

In the normal adult, the oxygen required for the work of respiration is about 1 to 2 percent of the total oxygen consumption. After open-heart surgery, the oxygen cost is increased to 10 to 50 percent of the total oxygen consumption, depending on the degree of pulmonary insufficiency [38]. Thus supplementary oxygen is needed in the immediate postoperative period. Children can usually be adequately managed by the administration of high humidity oxygen. Adults who have preexisting lung damage or alterations as a result of their surgical procedure will need respirator therapy.

Oxygen alone is inadequate because the central respiratory center is depressed by the anesthesia and drugs. Thus, the sole stimulation to respiration is the low oxygen tension, which stimulates the peripheral chemoreceptors. Administration of oxygen to the patient will raise the PO_2 and result in a decreased stimulus to the peripheral chemoreceptors. Although the PCO_2 may rise, it is often an inadequate stimulus to the depressed central respiratory center in the adult patient. Thus most cardiac surgeons feel that all open-heart surgery patients should have assisted respirations until the lungs are fully expanded, an adequate level of PO_2 can be maintained, and stabilization of the blood pressure, acid-base balance, blood volume, and vascular tone has taken place. Although the arterial carbon dioxide tension can be reduced by the proper use of a respirator, metabolic alkalosis may result if the blood bicarbonate is not also reduced, since the pH of the blood is determined by the ratio of the blood bicarbonate to the PCO_2 (Henderson-Hasselbalch equation). Some surgeons give a drug like acetazolamide (Diamox) which inhibits the enzymatic action of carbonic anhydrase in the formation of carbonic acid and promotes bicarbonate diuresis [29].

Types of Respirators

Negative-pressure Respirators

These respirators do not raise the mean intrapleural pressure (and thus the central venous pressure), so their use does not require the patient to increase his peripheral venous pressure to reconstitute the venous gradient to return blood to the heart [40]. The iron lung and electrophrenic respiration are types of negative-pressure respirators.

Electrophrenic respiration is rhythmic electrical stimulation of one phrenic nerve in the neck to increase the negativity of the intrapleural pressure and thereby cause the diaphragm to contract. It has been recommended by some surgeons for the patient who, because of hemorrhagic shock, has a lowered capacity for increasing his peripheral venous pressure. Most physicians feel that advocates of the use of electrophrenic stimulation to provide negative-pressure respiration have not adequately tested their theories.

Positive-pressure Respirators

These increase the mean intrapleural pressure and thereby decrease the cardiac output by impairing return of venous blood to the heart. This also stimulates compensatory arteriolar constriction. When the inspiratory time (during which the positive pressure is applied) is shorter than the expiratory time (during which no positive pressure is applied), the deleterious effects on the circulation are minimal. The ratio mentioned previously of 1:2 for inspiratory to expiratory time is recommended. Thus respirators that can be regulated to deliver positive pressure during only a short period of the total respiratory cycle keep the mean airway pressure low and are advantageous.

Patients on continuous respirator therapy should have a cuffed endotracheal tube or a cuffed tracheostomy tube. Because of the danger of infection in a patient who has had a sternum-splitting incision with destruction of the fascia barrier, tracheostomy is usually contraindicated in these patients. Patients can tolerate an endotracheal tube for 1 to 2 weeks if it is cared for properly.

There are two main types of positive-pressure respirators: pressure-cycled and volume-cycled.

Pressure-cycled Respirators

These respirators deliver air into the lungs until a preset pressure is reached, at which point the inspiratory phase stops and the expiratory phase begins. The volume of air that is delivered to the lungs depends on airway resistance, pulmonary compliance, and the rate of flow during the period of inspiration. These respirators cannot compensate for increased airway resistance. When resistance is increased the preset limit of pressure is reached more rapidly and the inspiratory period becomes very short. If the resistance is great, the machine will cycle rapidly—giving respiratory rates of 40 to 50/min—but it will deliver such a low tidal volume that only the dead space is ventilated.

The two main pressure-cycled respirators in use are the *Bennett* and the *Bird*. They can be used for intermittent treatment or for continuous respirator therapy. Most models have a timing mechanism to allow initiating inspiration automatically. Thus they can be used to control as well as to assist ventilation, although most patients need to be sedated before their respirations can be taken over completely.

The Bennett respirator is one of the simplest respirators to use and is less expensive in cost. Most models have a flow-sensitive pressure valve that slows the flow of gas to the patient when the preset limit of pressure has almost been reached. The inspiratory phase ends when the pressure is reached, and the passive expiratory phase begins. The expiratory period is terminated when the subatmospheric pressure initiated by the patient's effort to inspire trips the machine.

The Bird respirator, which is available in several different models, is more complex than the Bennett and is generally felt to be more satisfactory for a patient with respiratory insufficiency. A pressure-sensitive cutoff valve terminates inspiration when the preset limit of pressure is reached. A rapid respiratory rate can sometimes be controlled by moving the sensitivity lever to 20, which requires the patient to make a greater inspiratory effort to trigger the machine. Decreasing the inspiratory flow rate may also slow the respiratory rate. However, decreasing the flow rate may prolong the inspiratory period and result in a ratio of inspiratory to expiratory time that has deleterious effects on the circulation.

Nursing Management of a Patient on a Pressure-cycled Respirator

- Measure the tidal volume with a respirometer at least every hour to ensure that an adequate volume is delivered.

- Provide at least 15 cm H_2O pressure to produce an adequate tidal volume. In patients with reduced compliance, use higher pressures.

- Correct any leak in the system or the machine will either fail to cycle or the inspiration period will be overly prolonged if the cycling pressure is only reached after a period of time.

- Synchronize the patient's respirations with the machine, or the patient will "lead" the machine and may develop sub-atmospheric intrathoracic pressure while the apparatus is delivering positive mouth pressure (pressure above atmospheric level). This competition with the respirator increases the work of respiration.

- Humidification of the inspired gases is essential. Keep saline, or medication as ordered, in the nebulizer at all times. Utilize a slow-drip setup with IV tubing to avoid frequent refilling of the small nebulizer chamber. To provide more efficient humidification, use an in-line nebulizer with a heating element.

- Provide intermittent hyperinflation of the lungs by "sighing" the patient for 2 or 3 respirations per minute. When the pressure is momentarily increased to 30 cm H_2O, deeper and prolonged respiration will result. On the Bird machine, prolonging the inspiratory period by holding in the red pin near the sensitivity dial for 5 sec will also result in the delivery of a greater volume of air to the lungs.

- Since the mechanical properties of the airways can be affected by so many conditions (obstruction by a mucus plug, leak in the system, broncheolar spasm, and so on), check the minute alveolar volume and the blood gases frequently for patients on pressure-cycled respirators.

Volume-cycled Respirators

Most physicians feel that it is almost impossible with pressure-cycled respirators to maintain an adequate alveolar volume in a patient who has severe respiratory problems. Thus volume-cycled respirators are used for open-heart surgery patients who have had a prolonged bypass procedure or who have limited respiratory and/or myocardial reserve.

Volume-cycled respirators deliver a preset volume of air with each inspiration. The rate of respiration is usually set at 16 to 18 per minute. The amount of pressure exerted depends on the airway resistance and pulmonary compliance of the patient. The main advantages of volume-cycled respirators are:

1 Maintenance of a relatively stable minute volume regardless of changes in the mechanical properties of the lungs.

2 Operation with either room air or with air and oxygen mixture depending on patient's need for mechanical ventilation and/or oxygenation.

3 Control of ratio between inspiration-expiration time, with inspiration usually requiring only one-third of the time cycle. This prevents significant impairment of cardiac function.

There are a number of volume-cycled respirators available. It is impossible to give adequate information about each unit. Since changes are constantly occurring, the nurse and the physician need to make an intensive study of any machine they are using. The most sophisticated unit is worthless unless the staff thoroughly understands the physical setup and the principles that guide its use.

Following is a brief description of the more frequently used volume respirators, with a detailed description of the Engstrom.

The *air-shields* is a reasonably priced unit. It has a nebulizer attachment and an airway pressure gauge. If a limit on the pressure is preset, a monitor system will generate an alarm.

The *Emerson* respirator can be used with either an uncuffed or a cuffed endotracheal or tracheostomy tube. It has an automatic sighing mechanism that momentarily increases the tidal volume being delivered 9 or 10 times an hour. An alarm is given if a leak develops in the tubing. A "bleed-off" valve prevents the pressure from going over 45 cm H_2O. If the angle of the tubing going toward the patient is greater than 45 degrees, condensation will build up in the tubing.

The *Morch* respirator is the only volume respirator that cannot operate with a cuffed tube. When the pressure necessary to deliver the preset volume of gas has built up to the limit of pulmonary compliance, the remaining volume of gas will be vented around the tracheostomy tube carrying secretions upward into the pharynx where they can be expectorated or easily suctioned. Early models of this unit did not provide adequate humidity and necessitated the addition of a nebulizer. Later models have a heated nebulizer with a water trap to prevent water from condensing in the tubing. In contrast to other volume respirators, there is no pressure gauge and no control over inspiratory-expiratory ratios. The unit frequently produces respiratory alkalosis, necessitating the use of some CO_2 in the inspired air. It is not used frequently for open-heart surgery patients, but is used more often for crushing injuries of the chest.

The *Bird Mark VI* may be connected to the Mark XIV, but it is rather a complex machine to operate, with a poor system for humidification and an inadequate system to measure expired minute volume.

The *Bennett Volume MA-1* has been improved with a resultant increase in its use. It can be utilized to assist the patient's respiratory efforts or to control them. It has both adjustable volume and maximum pressure controls (to a maximum of 80 cm H_2O pressure on the new machines). The volume control is set for the desired tidal volume rather than for the minute ventilation. It has a built-in sigh mechanism, with control knobs for both volume and pressure limits for the sigh. When the desired volume cannot be given within the limits set for the pressure on either the respiration or the sigh, a signal is activated. Alarms are also given if the oxygen source is deficient, if the ratio of inspiration to expiration is more than 1:1, or if a preset tidal volume is not delivered. It has an efficient system for heated humidification, with the temperature of the water vapor kept at the patient's body temperature so nearly 100 percent humidified air is delivered to the alveoli. It also has a bacterial filter that limits contamination of the unit from another patient or from the air supply. The filters can be safely autoclaved between patients (Fig. 5–5).

The *Engstrom* respirator appears more complex and it is probably the most expensive of all the respirators. It is generally recognized as the most effective for the critical patient, since it can be relied upon to ventilate both lungs equally without giving dissimilar gas mixtures. Although the operation of the unit seems intricate at first, it is rather quickly mastered. Some of the main factors are:

1   It has a spirometer that measures the expired volume, from which the expired minute alveolar volume can be computed. If the

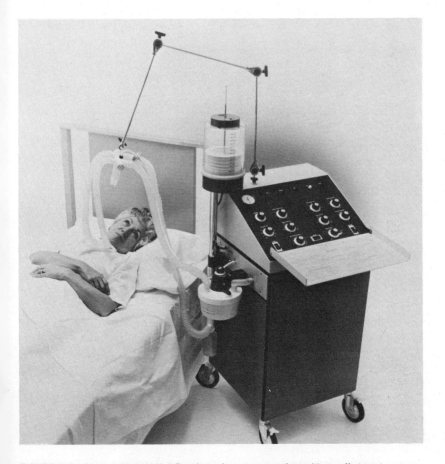

FIGURE 5–5   Bennett Model MA-1 Respirator in use on a patient with a cuffed tracheostomy. *(Photograph courtesy of Bennett Respiration Products, Inc., Santa Monica, Calif.)*

expired volume measured for a minute on the spirometer is different from the set volume, look for a leak in the system and either correct it or compensate for it by setting the delivered volume higher.

2   With each respiration, the actual pressure required to deliver the preset volume of air can be read on a pressure gauge. Sudden changes in pressure alert the nurse to the possibility of obstruction caused by a kink in the tubing, a plug in the airway, struggling of the patient, or other causes.

3   A water-trap valve acts to prevent pressures in excess of a predetermined amount. Pressures less than 35 cm H_2O are set by filling the water trap to the height of the desired pressure. With the water trap on, a pressure higher than 35 cm H_2O will not be delivered, but the excess volume will "bubble out" in the water trap. This bubbling in the water trap is easily noticed by personnel and yet it does not frighten the patient as an alarm would. The position of the water-trap valve can be reversed (or inverted), in which case there will not be any bubbling until the pressure exceeds 70 cm H_2O. For the few patients who need ventilatory pressures in excess of 70 cm H_2O, the water trap can be completely shut off. This patient would need to be observed extremely closely, since all pressure limits have been bypassed.

4   When the patient takes in small amounts of air between respirations, it will be recorded by the machine on the pressure gauge so early action can be taken before the patient is actively "fighting" the machine.

5   The unit has an adequate system for supplying humidity. It consists of a cylinder for tepid water with a sponge rubber insert. The pores in the sponge rubber increase the evaporation surface of the water and the water vapor is then carried along by the inspired gas to the patient. This provides approximately 100 percent humidity at room temperature, but when the air is warmed up by the heat of the body, the relative humidity drops to about 44 percent. To maintain the humidification system of the Engstrom at its optimum functioning, the nurse needs to:

(a) Soak any new sponges in detergent and water to reduce the surface tension that might keep them from absorbing water.

(b) Keep the sponge at the very top of the cylinder. Otherwise air entering the cylinder can flow across the top of the cylinder above the sponge and pass on out to the patient without being humidified.

(*c*) Maintain the proper level (as indicated on the gauge) of distilled tepid water in the cylinder at all times.

(*d*) Empty the condensed water container on the expiratory line regularly.

6 The machine is supplied with an extra inspiratory valve, which allows the patient to draw in a larger volume of air than is set by the machine. This valve is helpful in weaning the patient from the machine, as the staff can gradually reduce the volume settings and allow the patient to take the additional volume he needs from the atmosphere. It should usually be closed when attempting to synchronize the patient with the respirator so he cannot take extra breaths between respirations.

7 Unfortunately the respirator has no alarm system to warn the nurse that it has become disconnected from the patient, so the nurse needs to be in constant attendance. An Ambu bag should be attached to the machine to be used in case of mechanical failure.

Nursing Assessment   The effectiveness of the management of a patient on continuous volume-controlled respirator therapy depends on accurate nursing assessment with the identification of any problem and implementation of appropriate action.

• Observe synchronization of the patient's respirations with those of the respirator.

• Measure the expired minute volume at least once an hour and compare with the minute volume settings on the machine (or tidal volume measurements for machines that measure tidal volume rather than minute volume).

• Observe any sudden changes in airway pressures, and investigate possible causes.

• Identify any deviation from normal functioning of the respirator, especially as related to the system for humidification.

• Determine psychological response to respirator, and identify factors that enhance and those that hinder adjustment.

• Listen to the chest to determine flow of air to all areas.

• Evaluate laboratory determinations of blood gas studies.

Nursing Management of a Patient on a Volume-cycled Respirator   It is relatively easy to initiate the use of the respirator when the patient is placed on the unit immediately after surgery while he is still under the influence of anesthesia and sedation. To maintain him successfully on the respirator is a challenge to both the physician and the nurse.

Although nomograms are available to calculate the recommended initial volume settings for the patient based on his age and the surface area of his body, it has been found that a patient's respiratory function cannot be taken over completely in the early postoperative period without giving volumes at least 30 percent higher than predicted by the nomograms [41]. Machines are often set initially for adults at 6 liters air, 4 liters O_2, and 16 respirations per minute [36].

For most patients positive pressure is only given during the inspiratory phase of respiration. For patients with the shock-lung syndrome, *positive end expiratory pressure* (PEEP) has been recommended by some physicians. At the 44th Scientific Session of the American Heart Association, Dr. Henning Pontoppidan discussed his experience with the use of PEEP in the shock-lung syndrome. He found that the use of 5 cm water end expiratory pressure increased the lung volume and resulted in an improvement in oxygenation, a reduction in shunting, and an improvement in lung compliance. The main disadvantages are that raising the mean airway pressure increases the blood volume; the cardiac index may fall 10 to 15 percent; and the urine output may be decreased due to the increase in ADH hormone levels. A finding that has implications for nursing care is that when the pressure is removed abruptly, hypoxemia develops rapidly. Thus suctioning and anything else that requires removal from the respirator must be done in very short intervals of time.

Resynchronization of the patient to the respirator whenever he has been off the respirator for even a short period is sometimes difficult. If the patient has been suctioned or the endotracheal tube manipulated, the accompanying discomfort and apprehension may result in rapid, shallow respirations. Medication is sometimes required to suppress the patient's tachypneic respiratory effort. Narcotics or sedatives are frequently used. Some physicians use succinylcholine chloride (Anectine), or another similar muscle-relaxant drug. This drug is generally added to an intravenous infusion bottle with a microdrip and titrated at a rate to control the patient's respirations. Most physicians avoid using muscle relaxants whenever possible because of their potentially adverse effects on the circulatory function [40].

The author has found that patients can be resynchronized with the respirator with the use of very small amounts of intravenous morphine (3 to 5 mg every 2 hr) when their cooperation is elicited by means of the following technique:

Before the patient is hooked up to the respirator he is asked to listen to the machine and breathe in rhythm with the machine. The nurse verbally accents the rhythm by saying "in—and—out, in—and—out." If the patient has difficulty slowing his rate to that of the machine, light pressure on his chest with each "out" helps him to adjust to the rhythm. When the patient is breathing with the machine he is quickly reconnected during the expiratory period.

Some physicians recommend that patients be rapidly bagged (with an Ambu-type respirator bag) to the point of apnea, temporarily removing any stimulus to respiration before they are placed on the machine. The technique described above is not only more comfortable for the patient, but it answers the patient's need to have some control over his own situation.

If the patient's respirations cannot be synchronized through eliciting his cooperation and the giving of narcotics, the minute volume should be gradually increased and the water-trap valve inverted to allow pressures to the maximum of 70 cm H_2O. Sometimes volumes may temporarily exceed twice the value given on the nomogram. These adjustments are usually only made by the physician, and close observation of the patient during this period is absolutely essential.

If the patient's respiratory rate is 28, those with limited experience sometimes feel that increasing the rate of the respirator to 28 will result in synchronization. However, clinical trial has shown that this is not a satisfactory method of synchronizing the patient.

Regulating the controls to ensure adequate alveolar ventilation is done in response to blood gas reports. The first study should be made within 20 min of the initiation of respiratory therapy, with additional studies as indicated. Studies are usually done at least every 4 hr for the first 12 hr and then four times a day. Although the physician is usually responsible for ordering the volumes of oxygen and air, if he is not immediately available the nurse should not hesitate to adjust the volumes in response to a blood gas report. General principles for regulating volumes of inspired gases are:

1   The minute volume (total volume of room air and volume of oxygen delivered per minute) should not be increased or decreased more than two liters at a time.

2   The ratio of oxygen to room air delivered should not be greater than 80 percent. The deleterious effects of high oxygen concentrations have previously been described. Methods to increase humidification such as the use of an ultrasonic nebulizer attached to the respirator may result in less damage to the lungs if high concentrations for a short period are deemed essential for a patient. Table 5–2 shows the percent of oxygen that will be delivered with various combinations of volumes of air and oxygen. (Since room air contains 20 percent oxygen, the oxygen in the room air needs to be added to the pure oxygen to get the total percent of oxygen delivered.) The nurse does not usually set the controls at a level that delivers more than 80 percent oxygen.

3   In regulating the volumes of air and oxygen, it is necessary to look at all the figures and then interpret their meaning for the patient. Since the values may vary independently of each other, the minute volume and the ratio of oxygen to air must be individually adjusted.

(a) PO_2 is a measure of *oxygenation*. If the value is low, the concentration of oxygen is too low and the ratio of oxygen to air needs to be increased. This is accomplished by increasing the oxygen flow meter by 1 or 2 l/min and decreasing the room air volume by a like amount, maintaining the same minute volume. The patient's preoperative studies should be used as a guide to maintaining postoperative gas tension. The PO_2 is usually maintained about 10 to 30 percent above the preoperative level.

(b) PCO_2 is a measure of *ventilation*. An elevated PCO_2 means that the volume of ventilation is inadequate, and the total minute volume needs to be increased. A low PCO_2 means that the concentration of CO_2 is low because of hyperventilation, and the minute volume needs to be decreased. The minute volumes can be increased or decreased (usually in increments of 2 l/min) by referring to the table and selecting a setting that gives the same percentage of oxygen, but with altered minute volume. Thus if a hyperventilating patient has been on 12 liters of 50 percent oxygen he would have been receiving 4.5 liters O_2 and 7.5 liters air per minute. The setting would be changed to give a total of 10 liters of gas, of which 3.8 liters is oxygen and 6.2 liters is air. Many physicians believe that the minute volume should not be decreased below 10 and treat hypocapnia by adding rebreathing space

TABLE 5-2   OXYGEN-CONCENTRATION RATIOS

Total Minute Volume, liters	% Oxygen								
	20	30	40	50	60	70	80	90	100
15	15 air	1.8 O_2 / 13.2 A	3.9 O_2 / 11.1 A	5.6 O_2 / 9.4 A	7.5 O_2 / 7.5 A	9.3 O_2 / 5.7 A	11.2 O_2 / 3.8 A	13.0 O_2 / 2.0 A	15 O_2
14	14 air	1.7 O_2 / 12.3 A	3.6 O_2 / 10.4 A	5.2 O_2 / 8.8 A	7.0 O_2 / 7.0 A	8.7 O_2 / 5.3 A	10.5 O_2 / 3.5 A	12.2 O_2 / 1.8 A	14 O_2
13	13 air	1.6 O_2 / 11.4 A	3.3 O_2 / 9.7 A	4.9 O_2 / 8.1 A	6.5 O_2 / 6.5 A	8.1 O_2 / 4.9 A	9.7 O_2 / 3.3 A	11.3 O_2 / 1.7 A	13 O_2
12	12 air	1.5 O_2 / 10.5 A	3.1 O_2 / 8.9 A	4.5 O_2 / 7.5 A	6.0 O_2 / 6.0 A	7.5 O_2 / 4.5 A	9.0 O_2 / 3.0 A	10.5 O_2 / 1.5 A	12 O_2
11	11 air	1.4 O_2 / 9.6 A	2.8 O_2 / 8.2 A	4.2 O_2 / 6.8 A	5.5 O_2 / 5.5 A	6.9 O_2 / 4.1 A	8.2 O_2 / 2.8 A	9.6 O_2 / 1.4 A	11 O_2
10	10 air	1.3 O_2 / 8.7 A	2.5 O_2 / 7.5 A	3.8 O_2 / 6.2 A	5.0 O_2 / 5.0 A	6.3 O_2 / 3.7 A	7.5 O_2 / 2.5 A	8.8 O_2 / 1.2 A	10 O_2
9	9 air	1.2 O_2 / 7.8 A	2.3 O_2 / 6.7 A	3.4 O_2 / 5.6 A	4.5 O_2 / 4.5 A	5.7 O_2 / 3.3 A	6.7 O_2 / 2.3 A	7.9 O_2 / 1.1 A	9 O_2
8	8 air	1.1 O_2 / 6.9 A	2.0 O_2 / 6.0 A	3.1 O_2 / 4.9 A	4.0 O_2 / 4.0 A	5.0 O_2 / 3.0 A	6.0 O_2 / 2.0 A	7.1 O_2 / .9 A	8 O_2

between the ventilator and the patient to increase the dead space and keep the PCO_2 above 35 mm Hg [5].

(c) When a problem of ventilation exists with a problem of oxygenation, then both volume and gas ratios need to be adjusted.

The patient's adjustment to the respirator is facilitated when he has been prepared preoperatively for the experience and when he receives adequate emotional support.

Preoperative Preparation of the Patient

When the patient has been told before surgery that he will be on a respirator after surgery and will have a tube in his windpipe so he will not be able to talk, he remains calm as he emerges from anesthesia. Important aspects of the preoperative teaching are:

- Information about the reason for the use of the respirator.
- Explanation of the procedure he can expect in being removed from the machine, having his cuff deflated, secretions suctioned out, etc.
- Demonstration of the machine, with an opportunity for the patient to listen to the rhythm of the machine and practice breathing "in-and-out" with it. The patient should be allowed to choose whether or not he will visit the unit and look at the equipment. A few patients may use the defense mechanism of preferring to "take things as they come" as a method of avoiding a situation they feel will be too stressful for them.
- Opportunity to talk with another patient who has been maintained on a respirator is helpful.

Postoperative Support

This is most effective when the goal is to reduce anxiety and the feeling of powerlessness and includes:

- Frequent reinforcement of the information that the respirator is taking over the work of breathing so his heart can rest and have time to heal. Knowledge serves to reduce anxiety and fear.
- Explanation of what is going to be done before each time it is done, and asking the patient's permission to proceed helps to reduce the

feeling of powerlessness. It is difficult to give the patient any control in his immediate postoperative period, but the skillful nurse will see that this need is met by asking "I'm going to suction you now; Okay?" or "Do you think you need to be suctioned?"

- Demonstrating factors to the patient which he may not perceive himself that give reassurance. For example, pointing out that he is not dependent on the machine but can breathe on his own—and telling him when he is off the machine and breathing unassisted—reduces the anxiety and powerlessness he is experiencing.

- Provision for communication by giving the patient a magic slate for writing his needs and giving adequate time for him to relate his needs (Fig. 5–6). Sometimes it is difficult to determine the need because the patient cannot write clearly and questioning him fails to locate the problem. If the nurse seems hurried and responds that she doesn't understand what the patient is trying to tell her, he feels powerless to communicate his needs and his anxiety is understandably increased.

- Reminding the patient that the present situation is only temporary

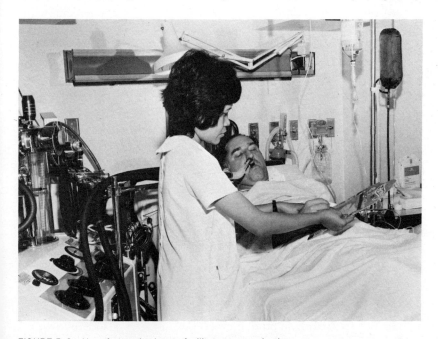

FIGURE 5–6 Use of a magic slate to facilitate communication.

helps the patient to be more tolerant of his condition. A remark such as "I'll bet you will be glad when you get that tube out so you can tell us what you're thinking" lets the patient know the nurse understands and accepts the way he feels.

Termination of Respirator Therapy

The decision that the patient can be safely removed from the respirator is usually based on the following criteria: (1) inspiratory pressure of 20 cm H_2O or less is required to deliver needed tidal volume, and (2) oxygen concentration can be decreased without adversely affecting the PO_2.

Measures to enhance satisfactory weaning from the respirator are:

- Leave the respirator on. The patient will usually continue to breathe in the same rhythm since he has become accustomed to it.

- Administer humidified and nebulized oxygen through the endotracheal tube by the use of a T adaptor on the end of the endotracheal tube. When the oxygen is connected to one end of the T crosspiece, the patient is able to exhale through the open end without having to exhale against the pressure of the flow of oxygen. If the patient has a tracheostomy, the nebulized oxygen can be given with a vented collar that fits loosely over the tracheostomy site. One-half normal saline is often used for nebulizers, since distilled water, which is hypotonic, is irritating to the mucous membranes.

- Discontinue all narcotics that depress respiration.

- Increase length of periods off the respirator from the initial 5 to 10 min/hr gradually, as tolerated. Ability to maintain a PO_2 of 70 or higher after being off the respirator for 30 min is usually an indication that the endotracheal tube is no longer needed. If intolerance for even short periods off the respirator is exhibited, weaning may have to be done by gradually decreasing the oxygen concentration until only room air is given. The volume of room air can then be gradually decreased if the respirator has an extra valve that permits the patient voluntarily to inspire additional room air. Some patients tolerate being off the respirator poorly because the blood-brain barrier is freely permeable to carbon dioxide but relatively impermeable to hydrogen and bicarbonate ions. Thus cerebrospinal fluid bicarbonate concentration may lag considerably behind arterial bicarbonate and cause a depression in respiration.

Periodically checking the blood gases for at least 48 hr after removal from the respirator should be done to detect delayed hypoventilation or hypoxia.

Intermittent positive pressure breathing (IPPB) treatments are usually given for 10- to 15-min periods every 4 hr, starting with the removal from the respirator. Opportunity to practice preoperatively usually increases the benefits received. The patient needs to be encouraged to: take a long, slow inspiration, hold an apneustic pause (pause at peak of inspiration), exhale slowly and completely, and cough after treatment is completed.

Some physicians are beginning to question the effectiveness of IPPB treatments in preventing pulmonary complications. One study found the incidence of pulmonary complications was actually in-

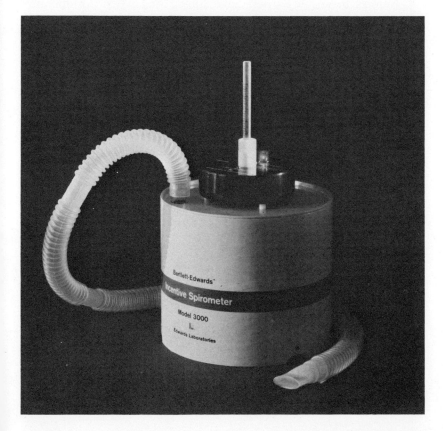

FIGURE 5-7   Incentive Spirometer to help the patient increase his lung capacity. *(Photograph courtesy of Edwards Laboratories, Santa Ana, Calif.)*

creased with IPPB, with the major causative factor identified as inadequate volume [42]. Other efforts to accomplish periodic hyperventilation have utilized rebreathing through a dead space or carbon dioxide inhalation. Although theoretically this should result in deeper respirations, in practice the respiratory rate has also increased, so large sustained volumes have not been achieved and rebreathing has not been found effective in reversing atelectasis [43].

Many methods have also been used to increase the expiratory period of respiration. The more frequently used ones provide some expiratory resistance as using blow bottles or blowing into a rubber glove or balloon. Since these maneuvers all result in intrapleural pressure higher than airway pressure (which could result in alveolar collapse), their effectiveness is also questioned [5].

Studies made by Bartlett have shown that when postoperative patients used voluntary sustained maximal inspiration with the glottis open (the maneuver was termed a "yawn") several times each hour, the findings of decreased lung volumes and transpulmonary shunting were markedly decreased [44]. A device that is termed an "incentive spirometer" or popularly called a "yawn box" is being tested on some surgical patients [5]. The instrument is preset for the desired inspiratory volume. Then the patient inhales through a tube until the light goes on, at which point he can exhale. Since he is inhaling through the tube his glottis will remain open so his intrapleural pressure will not be increased (Fig. 5–7).

Other methods of preventing atelectasis and shunting are in the process of being developed. The common elements uniting all devices that are successful in assisting ventilation are proper use and careful patient monitoring to see that the desired effect is being achieved.

NURSING MEASURES TO PROMOTE ADEQUATE RESPIRATION IN THE POSTOPERATIVE PERIOD FOR A PATIENT WITH AN ENDOTRACHEAL TUBE

Measures	Rationale
Secure the tube in place by tying with twill-type tape.	If the tube is allowed to slip into the right or left bronchus, one lung will not be adequately oxygenated. An unsecured tube can be pulled out by patient movement.
Keep the cuff inflated except for 2 to 5 min each hour when the cuff is deflated. Do not inflate cuff more than is necessary to prevent air from leaking around it when on the respirator.	Inflation helps maintain the proper position of the tube and prevents any vomitus from being aspirated. It is necessary to have a closed system when the patient is on the respirator, but pressure necrosis can develop unless pressure is released periodically to allow a good blood supply to the tissues.

NURSING MEASURES TO PROMOTE ADEQUATE RESPIRATION IN THE POSTOPERATIVE PERIOD FOR A PATIENT WITH AN ENDOTRACHEAL TUBE *(Continued)*

Measures	Rationale
Remove secretions by careful suctioning, using aseptic technique. (Guidelines for suctioning are in Appendix C.)	Airway must be kept patent for gaseous exchange to take place. Any mucus that decreases or obstructs the lumen of the respiratory passages contributes to atelectasis as the air distal to the occlusion is forced into the blood stream, resulting in the collapse of the alveoli [5]. Infection can be introduced into the distal airway by the suctioning catheter, expecially when there is damage to the mucosa.
Use an oral airway with an oral endotracheal tube for patients that are unresponsive to keep them from biting on the endotracheal tube.	Anything that narrows the lumen of the tube causes an obstruction to the flow of air.
Keep the endotracheal tube and the tubing to the respirator adequately supported.	Weight of tubing on the patient's mouth or nose can cause discomfort and pressure sores.
Use a folded bath blanket under the head in place of a pillow.	Flexion of the neck by a pillow can reduce the patency of the airway.
Provide adequate humidification of inspired gases when off the respirator. Heated nebulizers with ¾-in. tubing are usually utilized.	The natural humidifying mechanisms of the oral and nasopharynx are lost with intubation or tracheostomy. The usual oxygen bubbler setup with small bore tubing supplies only 7 to 20 percent humidity to the patient. Nebulizers supply a mist that can be carried along by the inspired gas into the lungs. Humidity varies with temperature, so nebulized gas that contains 100 percent humidity at room temperature will only contain approximately 44 percent humidity after it is warmed to the patient's body temperature. The use of ¾-in. tubing prevents compression of the gas which results in greater "rain-out" (droplets of moisture joining together and falling out of the suspension).
Use ultrasonic nebulization if more humidity is needed, expecially when high concentrations of oxygen are given.	Because it supplies small and uniform water molecules, the mist does not "rain-out" in the tubing or upper airways, but is carried to the distal alveoli. Advantages are better hydration of the pulmonary membrane, thinning of secretions, and maintenance of the ciliary action of the mucosa which helps the mucous secretions to be carried upward where they can be suctioned or coughed out.
Drain condensed moisture from tubing frequently.	Water droplets along the tubing result in more water condensation. Water in tubing can be inadvertently delivered to the patient.
Use a T piece (commonly called a "chimney") on the end of the endotracheal tube when delivering nebulized gas (Fig. 5–8).	This provides an expiratory port.

NURSING MEASURES TO PROMOTE ADEQUATE RESPIRATION IN THE POSTOPERATIVE PERIOD FOR A PATIENT WITH AN ENDOTRACHEAL TUBE *(Continued)*

Measures	Rationale
Unless sodium is restricted use half normal saline in the nebulizer chamber.	Irritation of the respiratory mucosa is minimal when isotonic solutions are used.
Add medication to the nebulizer only when secretions are very tenacious and thick.	Medications to reduce the surface tension of the alveoli are of little value except in cases of thick secretions [45].
Send a culture of tracheal secretions daily, or when there is a change in the character and amount of secretions. A sterile suction catheter with an attached specimen tube reduces contamination from other sources.	Early detection of infection increases effectiveness of treatment.
Send humidifiers and tubing for resterilization every 24 hr.	The warm, moist area provides a good media for bacterial growth.

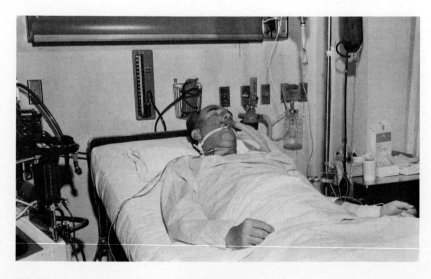

FIGURE 5–8   The use of a T piece on an endotracheal tube.

NURSING MEASURES TO PROMOTE ADEQUATE RESPIRATION IN THE POSTOPERATIVE
PERIOD AFTER EXTUBATION

Measures	Rationale
Inform the patient before his endotracheal tube is removed that he may have some hoarseness and a sore throat which should only be temporary.	Advance knowledge reduces anxiety that accompanies adjustment to adverse situations.
Observe closely after extubation for edema of the larynx and trachea.	Edema is usually temporary, but severe edema can develop several hours or even days after removal of the tube. Severe edema may necessitate a tracheostomy. Large doses of steroids are sometimes needed to decrease severe edema.
Administer high humidity air or air and oxygen mixture by ¾-in. tubing with a face mask.	Humidified gas helps prevent edema and keeps secretions loose so they can be easily coughed up.
Turn the patient every 1 or 2 hr.	Frequent turning and movement help to equilibrate ventilation and perfusion in all areas of the lungs and thus aid in lung expansion [5].
Assist patient to hyperinflate his lungs for at least 3 to 5 respirations every 1 or 2 hr, using IPPB, blow bottles, or a "yawn box." Test expired volume with a respirometer when IPPB is used (Fig. 5–9).	With deep inspiration the intrathoracic pressure falls, which increases the return of blood to the right atrium. Periodic maximal inflation is essential to prevent atelectasis. A decrease in body activity will result in loss of muscle tone, with decreased ability to expand lungs. Unless the expired volume is measured, it is impossible to tell if the IPPB treatment has resulted in inflation to total lung capacity. Blow bottle volume can be measured on the bottle, but it is not as satisfactory since it results in an intrapleural pressure higher than the airway pressure, which predisposes to alveolar collapse [5]. "Yawn-box" (incentive spirometer) looks promising but it is still in the testing stage [5].
Sit the patient up and provide firm support over the incisional area while he takes several deep breaths using the abdominal muscles and then coughs on expiration.	Retained secretions lead to pneumonia and atelectasis. Use of abdominal muscles in respiration increases volume of inspired air and helps to open the alveoli.
Use ultrasonic nebulizers if unable to raise secretions.	Penetration of the mist to the distal alveoli helps to thin secretions and maintain the ciliary action of the mucosa so secretions are carried upward and can be coughed out.
Alternate encouragement and assistance to coughing, with periods of rest.	Better patient cooperation is secured when the patient is allowed to rest and then mobilize his forces for the effort.

NURSING MEASURES TO PROMOTE ADEQUATE RESPIRATION IN THE POSTOPERATIVE
PERIOD AFTER EXTUBATION *(Continued)*

Measures	Rationale
If all efforts to get patient to cooperate in coughing fail, remove secretions by tracheal suctioning with a nasally passed catheter.	Uncomfortable procedures increase the patient's stress and should only be undertaken when all other methods fail.
If coughing is ineffective in preventing atelectasis and pneumonia, use postural drainage with vibrating and clapping techniques to promote drainage of secretions.	In order to drain the lung adequately, the position of the patient must be specific for the area to be drained. A physical therapist or a nurse with special training and practice is needed for the clapping and vibrating techniques. The percussive action produced by clapping dislodges plugs of mucus, allowing air in the lungs to penetrate behind the secretions and help move them toward the main bronchi and trachea [46].
Encourage leg exercises and early ambulation.	Bed rest limits lung excursion and results in loss of tone of respiratory and other muscles of the body.
Detect early signs of gastric distension and use a nasogastric tube to provide decompression.	Gastric distension inhibits lung expansion and may result in vomiting and aspiration.
Listen to the chest with a stethoscope for such sounds as stridor, wheezing, or labored ventilation that may mean presence of bronchospasm. Prompt treatment should include the identification of any possible allergen and the use of aerosolized and systemic bronchodilators, sedation, and, if severe, corticosteroids.	Any spasm of the bronchus limits flow of gas to periphery of the lung. Cause is frequently an allergen, pulmonary edema, or underlying chronic obstructive pulmonary disease.

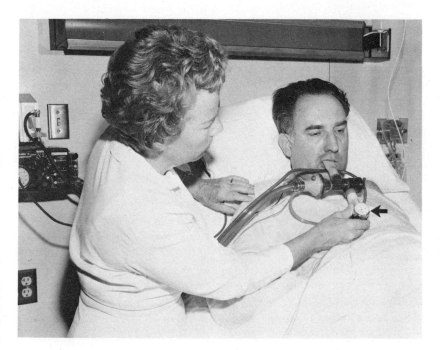

FIGURE 5-9   A respirometer is connected to the exhalation port of IPPB tubing to measure the tidal volume. Usually 10 respirations are measured and the total divided by 10 to get the average tidal volume.

NURSING MEASURES TO PROMOTE GOOD EXPANSION OF THE LUNGS IN THE POSTOPERATIVE PERIOD FOR A PATIENT WITH CHEST TUBES

Measures	Rationale
Connect the tubes to an airtight drainage system such as water seal drainage or a unit with a flutter-type valve.	By draining the chest cavity of accumulated blood or air that might leak from the lung surface, the negative intrapleural pressure necessary for reexpansion of the lungs is restored. (Both water seal and flutter valves act as one-way valves permitting air to escape on expiration but preventing air from entering with inspiration.) Water seal drainage must be connected so that the tubing from the patient is connected to the glass tube with the distal portion submerged in water.
If suction is used, check pressure gauge on machine to ensure maintenance of proper pressure level.	15- to 20-cm H_2O negative pressure facilitates drainage.
Observe and record color and amount of drainage hourly, keeping a	Color indicates whether bleeding is active or old. Blood loss is usually replaced volume for volume. It is essential to know whether replacement is ahead or behind at all times.

NURSING MEASURES TO PROMOTE GOOD EXPANSION OF THE LUNGS IN THE
POSTOPERATIVE PERIOD FOR A PATIENT WITH CHEST TUBES *(Continued)*

Measures	Rationale
cumulative record of the blood balance. An adhesive strip up the bottle provides a convenient method of marking the level. Report any sudden rise.	
Investigate any cessation of flow of blood that may indicate a clot, obstruction, or kink in the tubing.	If flow is obstructed, blood can collect in the chest and cause collapse of the lung. The physician may need to be called to irrigate the tube.
Observe level of fluid in drainage tubing for fluctuation. In immediate postoperative period, the level should rise with inspiration.	The negative pressure in the intrapleural space increases with inspiration, pulling fluid in the tubing toward the lung. When lung is fully expanded, noticeable fluctuation ceases.
"Strip" or "milk" the chest tubes every hour for the entire length of the tubing.	Compression of the tube helps dislodge clots and maintain patency. Since only air usually drains through the top tube, it may only be necessary to milk the bottom tube.
Use the following safety measures to prevent air from entering the lungs: 1. Keep two clamps at bedside to clamp off tubes if the bottle or water seal is broken. 2. Tape all connections to prevent unintentional separation. 3. Keep bottles in a caddy or tape them to the floor to prevent them from being accidentally kicked.	If air is allowed to enter the thoracic cavity, it could cause a pneumothorax. Keeping the chest bottles in a caddy or taped to the floor also keeps them from being raised higher than the patient's chest, which could result in backflow of liquid into the lungs.
Keep tube positioned so it is in a continuous downward direction without kinks. Secure to bed, allowing adequate slack to accommodate turning.	Drainage is facilitated when flow is in a downward direction. Properly securing the tube helps prevent having the tube pulled out prematurely.

NURSING MEASURES TO PROMOTE GOOD EXPANSION OF THE LUNGS IN THE
POSTOPERATIVE PERIOD FOR A PATIENT WITH CHEST TUBES *(Continued)*

Measures	Rationale
Change chest drainage bottle when it is three-fourths full. Two persons should work together and double-clamp tubes proximally to the patient before they are separated from the old suction tubing.	Two persons are necessary to prevent contamination and ensure patient safety.
Assist both patient and physician when chest tubes are removed.	Chest tubes are usually removed after 24 to 48 hr if lung is expanded, bleeding has ceased, and there is no air leak. Suction is maintained in tube while it is being removed, and the patient is instructed to take a deep breath and hold it while the tube is being removed.
After chest tubes are removed, inspect the pressure dressing frequently and reinforce as necessary.	Pressure dressing is kept on for 12 to 24 hr to prevent excessive bleeding and keep air from entering thoracic cavity.

THE CARDIOVASCULAR SYSTEM

6

PHYSIOLOGY

The human adult heart is about the size of a closed fist. It is composed of three layers: the endocardium, myocardium, and epicardium. It is enclosed in a double-walled sac, the pericardium. The heart has four chambers. The upper chambers (atria) receive the blood and are thin-walled. The lower chambers (ventricles) pump the blood and have thicker walls. The wall of the left ventricle is the thickest of all the chambers, being three times as thick as the wall of the right ventricle. The rounded apex of the heart is formed by the left ventricle and is just behind the sixth rib, about three inches to the left of the sternum. The smaller right ventricle does not extend as far as the left ventricle. The left atrium is almost vertically above the right atrium, so that the two atria form a vertical axis behind the sternum, and the two ventricles slope off slightly to the left [47] (Fig. 6–1).

The superior and inferior venae cavae bring the blood from the body to the right atrium. During ventricular diastole (relaxation) blood passes through the tricuspid valve into the right ventricle. During ventricular systole (contraction) the tricuspid valve closes and the blood in the right ventricle passes out

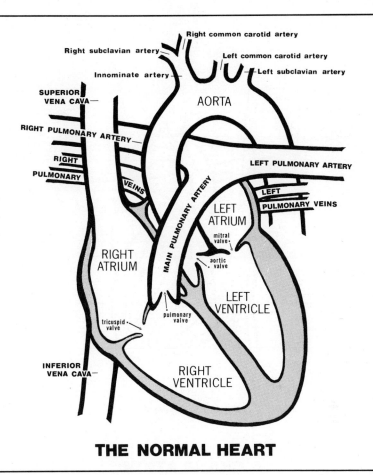

THE NORMAL HEART

FIGURE 6–1

through the pulmonary valve into the pulmonary artery and to the lungs. While in the lungs the blood gives off carbon dioxide and picks up oxygen. The oxygenated blood then reaches the left atrium through the four pulmonary veins. During ventricular diastole it passes through the mitral valve, a bicuspid valve, into the left ventricle. In the ensuing ventricular systole, the mitral valve closes, the aortic valve opens, and the blood is forced out through the aortic valve into the aorta (Fig. 6–2). Ten percent of all the blood flows back through the coronary arteries, but the coronary flow is during diastole, not during systole. The force of the blood into the aorta

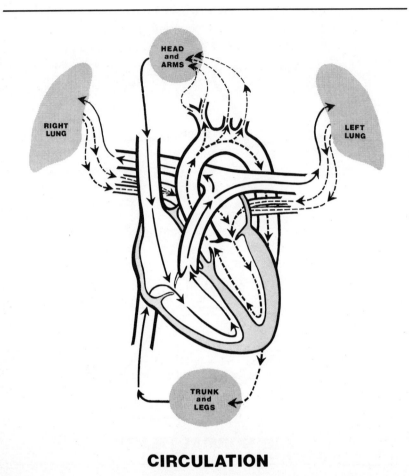

CIRCULATION

FIGURE 6–2 Diagram of the normal flow of blood. Unoxygenated blood is represented by solid lines; oxygenated blood is represented by dotted lines.

distends it and creates pressure within it. This pressure then pushes the blood through the arteries, arterioles, capillaries, veins, and finally back into the heart. The small arteries, arterioles, capillaries, and small veins have such small diameters that blood flows through them only with considerable difficulty. The vessels offer resistance to the flow of blood.

Adequate circulation depends on an effective combination of cardiac pump, blood volume, and vascular tone [48].

The Heart as a Pump

The heart is composed of muscle fibers, and many physiologists consider it to be a syncytium (a network of cells lacking separate cell membranes). The membrane is thick in places forming intercalated disks that are probably sites of enzyme concentration, assisting in the rapid conduction of the impulse for contraction (rate is 800 cm/sec) [47].

The atria and the ventricles contract sequentially. First the atria and then the ventricles contract. The right and left sides of the heart function independently of each other, but they operate simultaneously. The rhythmical electrical impulse for contraction (depolarization) in the normal heart is initiated and regulated by the sinoatrial node located in the right atrium. Each contraction of the atria is followed by a period of repolarization (sometimes referred to as "recharging"), which occurs while the ventricles are contracting and becoming depolarized. The ventricular contraction is followed by a period of recovery while the cells become repolarized and the chambers fill with blood. The cardiac cycle is thus composed of periods of depolarization and repolarization characterized by specific electrical activity. However, the heart can depolarize without any muscular contraction taking place. Only the muscular "pumping" activity of the heart will be considered now; in a later section measurement of the electrical activity of the heart by the electrocardiograph tracing will be discussed.

The *cardiac output* is the amount of blood pumped out of the left ventricle per minute. It is the product of the stroke volume (amount of blood pumped by the left ventricle with each contraction) and the heart rate. If the heart rate is 70/min and the stroke volume is 80 ml, the cardiac output would be 70×80 ml or 5600 ml/min. The total amount of blood pumped by the normal heart at rest is 5 l/min. During exercise it increases to 25 to 30 l/min or it can decrease to 1.5 l/min following hemorrhage.

Although there is now no accurate, reliable, and easily used device to measure cardiac output that does not alter the function being measured, a radioisotope dilution technique using precordial detection of the radioisotope indicator or the injection of indocyanine dye with measurement of the quantitative dilution curve are techniques occasionally employed. Electronic monitors, which show great promise for the future, are being developed. Some equipment being used experimentally includes the use of the aortic-pressure curve to give the stroke volume in real time, and the use of the change in thoracic impedance to yield both stroke volume and respiratory gas flow without penetrating the skin [49].

In the process of development are fiber-optic catheters that can be placed in arteries to measure the various wavelengths of reflected light and give continuous dye concentration recordings that potentially can be used for cardiac output, left ventricular diastolic volume, plasma volume, and liver function tests on one wavelength and hemoglobin concentration, percent oxygen saturation, and carboxyhemoglobin on others. If the selective light- and pressure-sensitive devices can be incorporated into a single fiber-optic catheter, it will result in more information while decreasing the number of lines and cables attached to the patient.

The *stroke volume* is the amount of blood pumped by the left ventricle with each contraction. The diastolic volume of the left ventricle equals the stroke volume except in cases of incomplete emptying when the volume of blood in the ventricle must be subtracted from the diastolic volume to obtain the stroke volume.

The distensibility and contractility of the ventricular walls represent changes in the physiologic condition of the myocardium and the degree of compliance affects the stroke volume. From studies made by Frank and Starling, it has been found that the myocardium can increase its force of contraction and thus its stroke volume by two major means:

1 Increasing the length of the muscle fiber from its original state (stretching of the fiber) by an increase in the volume of blood. However, above a certain point or in a failing heart, increasing the diastolic stretch will result in a diminution of the force of contraction.

2 Shifting the relationship between the force of the tension developed in the muscle fiber and the velocity of its contraction. Increased contractility is present only if the velocity of shortening is maintained while a greater load is applied [29].

When these principles are applied the following relationships are demonstrated:

1 The diastolic filling is determined by the effective filling pressure and the resistance to distension offered by the wall of the ventricle.

2 The amount of blood ejected during systole is affected by the blood pressure, blood volume, and the degree of myocardial shortening that can occur against that particular outflow pressure.

Adequate stroke volume also depends on competent heart valves that move freely and close completely to prevent regurgitation of blood.

The *heart rate* is increased or decreased as a result of changes in pressure on the receptors located in the wall of the arch of the aorta and the carotid sinus. These changes in pressure control the secretory activity of the sympathetic and parasympathetic nervous systems. The parasympathetic, also called the vagal, system secretes acetylcholine at the end of the nerve fibers. The sympathetic, also termed ganglionic or adrenergic, system secretes epinephrine and norepinephrine, which are termed catecholamines. The main actions of the two systems on the heart are:

1 The parasympathetic nerves; which *(a)* slow the atrial rate of the heart, *(b)* decrease the heart output, and *(c)* decrease the force of contraction of cardiac muscle.

2 The sympathetic nerves; which *(a)* increase the heart rate, *(b)* increase the heart output, *(c)* dilate the coronary arteries, resulting in increased blood flow, *(d)* increase the force of contraction of the cardiac muscle, and *(e)* increase splanchnic and peripheral vasoconstriction.

The term *sympathomimetic* has been given to the group of drugs that stimulate the sympathetic system. Since their action is on the postganglionic adrenergic nerves, they are also called *adrenergic* drugs. Drugs that block the sympathetic nervous system are called *sympatholytic* drugs. Drugs that act on the sympathetic system to stimulate the heart are called *cardiotonic* drugs. Cardiotonic drugs are further divided into drugs that increase the force of the heart's contraction, or *positive inotropic,* and drugs that increase the heart rate, or *chronotropic.*

Catecholamines and other sympathomimetic agents can cause either excitation or inhibition of smooth muscle, depending primarily on the site and to a lesser extent on the dose. Ahlquist [50] has divided the adrenergic receptors into two types: alpha (α) and beta (β). *α receptors* are the adrenoceptive sites on smooth muscles where catecholamines produce excitation. They are associated with vasoconstriction, myocardial ectopic excitation, intestinal relaxation, iris dilation, and muscle contraction. β *receptors* are the sites on the smooth muscle concerned with inhibition. They are associated with vasodilation, cardioacceleration, myocardial augmentation, and bronchial relaxation.

The heart has mainly β receptors, but the blood vessels have both α and β receptors. The choice of sympathomimetic drug to use depends on the desired action and desired site of the action. Appendix B contains a chart of the main cardiotonic drugs and their effect.

Drugs that stimulate the parasympathetic (vagus) nerves are termed *vagotonic,* and those that depress the vagus are termed *vagolytic.* Vagal stimulation will increase the vagal tone and is sometimes used to interrupt a supraventricular tachycardia. Since there are probably no vagal fibers to the ventricles, vagal stimulation has no effect on ventricular rate. Carotid sinus massage, gagging, and holding the breath are some of the methods used to stimulate the vagus. Since the bifurcation of the carotid artery is a common site of atherosclerotic plaques that may break off and go to the brain, carotid massage is usually only done by the physician. Atropine will block the vagal effect on the heart and thus increase the heart rate.

The heart rate is also affected by (1) changes in the temperature (cold slows the rate, heat to 40°C increases the rate and strength of the heart beat) and (2) the ionic constitution (the proper levels of sodium, calcium, potassium, and chloride are a necessity for normal rate).

Blood Volume

The normal adult blood volume is 5 to 6 l. Four-fifths of the blood is in the systemic circulation and one-fifth is in pulmonary circulation and the heart. Large veins of the abdominal region, venous sinuses of the liver, the spleen, venous plexuses of the skin, and pulmonary vessels act as storage places or reservoirs for blood. Should volume be lost from the vascular space, these reservoir veins contract and attempt to maintain venous pressure and diastolic cardiac filling. The relationship between the blood volume and the stroke volume has already been described. Normally an optimal blood volume provides adequate circulation with a minimum of cardiac work. When cardiovascular dynamics are impaired, the aim of blood volume management is to maintain a blood volume that will provide as adequate a circulation as the heart is capable of maintaining without risking cardiac decompensation by circulatory overloading.

Vascular Tone

The vascular tone is dependent on the capacity of the vascular system and its resistance. Normally the blood vessels dilate and contract. The amount of the resistance is generally dependent on:

1   The *length* of the vessel. The longer it is, the greater the resistance.

2   The *diameter* of the vessel. The smaller the diameter, the greater the resistance.

3   The *viscosity* of the fluid. The greater it is, the greater the resistance.

Man's ability to adapt to a wide variety of external conditions and internal metabolic states is due to a great extent to the adaptive ability of the peripheral circulation to meet the oxygen and nutrition needs of the cells. The mechanisms for adaptation are:

Autoregulation, or the ability of the tissues to increase their blood flow by local vasodilatation without the need for neural intercession. Local metabolites accumulating during ischemia may be responsible for this process [29].

Control by the autonomic nervous system. As previously stated, the degree of constriction of the smooth muscle in the walls of arterioles and veins is regulated to a major extent by the release of norepinephrine from the adrenergic or sympathetic nerve endings. A decrease in blood pressure stimulates vasoconstriction, which results in a decrease of capillary beds and is a homeostatic mechanism for maintaining the mean arterial pressure and normal flow of blood to the vital organs.

An *increase in the blood pressure* can cause reflex slowing of the heart through vagal stimulation and vasodilatation as acetylcholine is released, which then acts to effect a lowering of the blood pressure.

Electrical Activity of the Heart

The muscle cells of the heart have the capability of transmitting an impulse because of the electrical potential in their cell membrane. When the cell is in a resting state, its membrane will become positively charged. The negative ions, which equal the positive ions, will be within the cell, and the cell is said to be *polarized*. Neutrality exists between the positive ions (generally considered to be potassium ions) on the outside and negative ions inside the cell, but these cells have an intrinsic characteristic of becoming unstable. One positive ion enters the cell and the process of depolarization is started. The term *spontaneous discharge cycle* refers to the characteristic time during which the heart cells become charged, neutral, unstabilized, and discharged.

In the normal heart the electrical stimulus for depolarization starts in the sinoatrial (SA) node and the spontaneous discharge time is $1/60$ to $1/100$ min. Since the SA node controls the heart rate, it is called the pacemaker. (Although all areas of the myocardium may become initiators of the impulse, they only do so under abnormal conditions.)

From the SA node the stimulus travels like the waves of a pebble dropped into a pond throughout the atrial muscles, stimulating the atria to contract. The stimulus then, more slowly, crosses the atrioventricular (AV) node and passes down the bundle of His. It descends rapidly through the left and right bundle branches and spreads through the system of fibers over the inside of the ventricles called the Purkinje fibers (Fig. 6–3). The depolarization of the ventricles stimulates them to contract, after which there is a period of rest and then repolarization, which is the restoration of the membrane potential. After a chamber has been depolarized, it is refractory (resistant) to any additional stimulus to depolarization until it has become repolarized or "recharged." The refractory period has been divided into the absolute refractory period when it will not respond to any stimulus and the relative refractory period during which the membrane will respond, but only to an intense stimulus.

The electrical forces within the heart are transmitted outward and can be measured on the skin if electrodes are placed on the skin and attached to a galvanometer. An electrocardiograph (EKG) machine is a galvanometer with a device to record electrical activity. Recording is accomplished by a hot needle or stylus that melts the wax layer on a moving roll of paper, exposing the layer of carbon.

In order to view the electrical forces of the heart in all three of its dimensions, 12 leads (or planes) are used. In some instances it is helpful to explore additional higher and more lateral areas of the precordium. To help diagnose some abnormal patterns of heart conduction, an esophageal electrode may be used to obtain a tracing from behind the left atrium, or a transvenous wire electrode may be used to obtain a tracing from the cavity of the right atrium. The ultrasonic Doppler method of EKG study is sometimes used to detect an atrial beat that is impossible to detect with the usual EKG tracing [51].

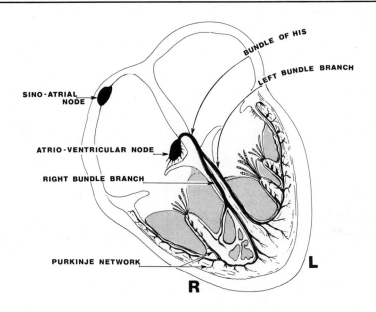

SINO-ATRIAL NODE

ATRIO-VENTRICULAR NODE

RIGHT BUNDLE BRANCH

PURKINJE NETWORK

BUNDLE OF HIS

LEFT BUNDLE BRANCH

L

R

CONDUCTION SYSTEM

FIGURE 6–3   Structures involved in the normal electrical conduction of the heart.

A complete circuit is necessary for electrocardiography. Each lead requires two electrodes, and the electrical activity of the heart travels a circuit from the heart, through one electrode to the electrocardiograph machine, through the other electrode, and back to the heart. In order for the electric current to flow, the voltage in one part of the circuit has to be higher than the voltage in the other part of the circuit. Each lead thus shows the difference in electrical potential of the two electrodes used for that lead.

The three standard limb leads are useful in the diagnosis of cardiac arrhythmias and in the determination of axis deviation. They are called bipolar leads because they show the activity of the heart as viewed simultaneously from two different locations. The electrodes may be placed on the extremities since the distance is infinite, but the electrical potential recorded is actually derived from the two shoulders and the left groin, with the heart approximately in the center of the triangle formed by the electrodes. The electrode picks up the electrical activity of the cardiac structures it faces, so the three standard leads view the activity of the heart from its lateral aspects. One disadvantage is that all three electrodes are in the frontal plane of the body, and do not adequately pick up the electrical activity of the anterior and posterior surfaces of the heart.

The three standard leads are taken after the electrodes are properly placed by turning the selection switch on the EKG machine:

Lead   I = left arm − right arm
Lead II = left leg − right arm
Lead III = left leg − left arm

Einthoven, who also designed the string galvanometer, established the polarity of the limb electrodes based on an equilateral triangle in which the sum of Lead I, Lead II, and Lead III equaled zero.

The greatest electrical potential comes from the left ventricle, since the muscle of the left ventricle is the thickest. Therefore the electrode on the left side below the diaphragm or on the left leg will be the most positive electrode. The left shoulder or arm has less electrical potential than the left leg. Thus it is negative in relation to the left leg, but positive in relation to the right arm or shoulder. The right shoulder has the least electrical potential because the normal current of flow of electricity is always away from the right shoulder, thus it is always negative compared with anything else.

The leads were set up so that most of the time in most people the QRS would be positive, that is, it would be above the baseline on the EKG paper. If an impulse is below the baseline, it is termed a negative deflection.

Another algebraic application of Einthoven's law is that a complex in Lead II is equal to the sum of the corresponding complexes in Leads I and III [52]. Thus if the QRS complex is upright in Leads I and III, Lead II will be as high as the two combined. Since Lead II has the most amplitude on the graph paper, it is generally considered to be the most informative of the limb leads. Monitoring equipment is sometimes limited to one lead, which is somewhat equivalent to Lead II if the electrodes are properly placed.

The three augmented unipolar limb leads help to eliminate the double exposure effect of the standard limb leads by recording the electrical activity as seen from one extremity only. They are of value primarily in determining if the findings of the Q wave on the standard lead were caused by cardiac position or by actual damage to the myocardium. The augmented unipolar limb leads measure the difference between the voltage picked up by an electrode on that extremity and the sum of the voltages as seen simultaneously by the other two limb electrodes:

aVL = left arm − (right arm + left leg)
aVR = right arm − (left arm + left leg)
aVF = left leg − (left arm + right arm)
where: L = left arm
R = right arm
F = left leg

The precordial leads give information about the anterior and posterior surfaces of the heart because an "exploring electrode" is placed on the anterior chest and then moved around the curve of the thorax to obtain views of the heart from different angles. The V leads, as the most commonly used precordial leads are called, are especially helpful in determining the location of a bundle branch block, and in the diagnosis of ventricular hypertrophy and myocardial infarction. They may also differentiate between ventricular ectopy and aberrance.

In the V precordial leads, the limb leads are all connected in a central terminal that has almost no electrical potential throughout the cardiac cycle. The central terminal is termed an indifferent electrode. The exploring electrode is thus the main determinant of the pattern, with each position standardized so that a certain cardiac structure is viewed in each lead. The locations of the exploring electrode in the six precordial leads usually used are:

V_1 The fourth intercostal space, just to the right of the sternum
V_2 The fourth intercostal space, just to the left of the sternum
V_3 Halfway between the positions of V_2 and V_4
V_4 The fifth intercostal space in the midclavicular line
V_5 The left anterior axillary line at the same level as V_4
V_6 The midaxillary line at the same level as V_4

EKG monitors have electronic filters to stabilize the baseline and attenuate 60-cycle noise. These filters may produce distortions, so conventional EKG tracings should be used for definitive therapy.

NURSING ASSESSMENT OF CARDIOVASCULAR PERFORMANCE

The maintenance of adequate circulation has been shown to depend on certain physiological and emotional factors. Careful observation of the patient's appearance and interpretation of data obtained from monitoring equipment, integrated with an adequate understanding of the underlying scientific and behavioral principles, form the basis for making a sound nursing diagnosis (see chart at end of chapter).

Arterial Blood Pressure

The pressure in a blood vessel is the force that the blood exerts against the walls of the vessel. This force is what makes blood continue to flow through the circulation. The blood pressure is mainly the result of two factors: cardiac output and peripheral resistance. Cardiac output has already been shown to be the product of the stroke volume and the heart rate; peripheral resistance is determined by the constriction and dilatation of the arterioles. The velocity and volume of flow in arteries is increased by increased cardiac output and decreased by increased resistance. In the human, the normal peak systolic pressure is about 120 mm Hg during each cycle and falls to a minimum diastolic pressure of about 70 mm Hg. There may be irreversible damage to the reticular system when the blood pressure is below 60 systolic for several hours. Cuff blood pressures can be measured with a cuff on the arms or the legs. Normally a cuff pressure from the leg is higher (as much as 30 mm Hg) than a cuff pressure taken from the arm.

The *pulse pressure* is the difference between systolic and diastolic pressure, which is normally about 50 mm Hg. It is narrowed in patients with a low blood pressure and a rapid heart rate because of the shortened diastolic emptying time.

The *mean pressure* is the average pressure throughout the cardiac cycle. Because systole is shorter than diastole, the mean pressure is slightly less than the value halfway between systolic and diastolic pressure. It can be determined by taking the diastolic pressure plus one-third of the pulse pressure. The mean pressure is frequently considered more meaningful in assessment than the systolic over the diastolic pressure.

When shock occurs, the compensatory mechanisms of vaso-constriction and arteriolar constriction may give a cuff blood pressure reading that is higher than the central pressure. With patients in shock who have a systolic blood pressure of below 90, cuff errors have been found to be as high as 30 percent. Thus central arterial pressure readings are preferred for postoperative cardiac patients and patients in shock. An additional advantage of central arterial pressures is that they can be read continuously and thus a change in the blood pressure can be immediately recognized.

The *central arterial pressure* is measured by a transducer, sometimes termed a strain gauge. It is an electromanometer, whereby mechanical energy is converted to electrical energy. The arterial pressure displaces a diaphragm in the gauge. The movement of the diaphragm puts "strain" on a thin wire in the gauge, and this changes the electrical resistance of the wire (Fig. 6–4). The blood pressure can either be read from a meter or from an oscilloscope. The oscilloscope records changes in electrical potential by means of a beam that sweeps across a screen. The screen has a grid that is calibrated to measure pressures. The closure of the aortic valve can also be observed on the waveform (Fig. 6–5).

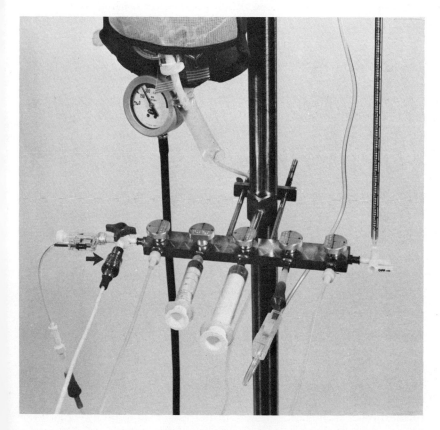

FIGURE 6–4 CENTRAL ARTERIAL PRESSURE MEASUREMENT The arrow points to the transducer, which measures the pressure. The use of a pressure infusor around a transfer pack unit filled with heparinized solution helps maintain a slow drip to keep the arterial line open. The rigid tubing to the right of the transducer connects to the patient's artery. Also shown to the far left is a CVP manometer. Blood may be drawn from the center ports for blood gas studies.

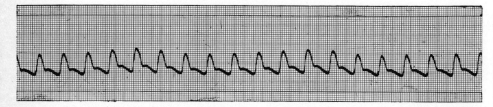

FIGURE 6–5 An arterial pulse wave obtained from a catheter in the brachial artery. The normal pulse wave is characterized by an initial, rather rapid anacrotic rise to a rounded peak or "anacrotic" shoulder. After the peak pressure is reached, the pressure falls gradually, making the descending limb of the pressure pulse wave less steep than the ascending limb. The descent is interrupted by the closure of the aortic valve (predicrotic notch), which results in a small rise in the pulse wave (dicrotic wave), followed by a gradual descent until the next ejection of blood from the ventricle.

To measure the arterial pressure, the transducer is connected to a Teflon catheter inserted in one of the main arteries. Any tubing between the transducer and the catheter must be rigid to prevent distortions of the readings caused by dissipation of pressure by the walls of the tubing. In order to avoid clotting of the blood in the line, a slow drip is maintained with a heparinized solution. A pump may be employed to maintain the arterial drip, but an easier method is to use a pressure infusor bag around a transfer blood pack unit. If the sphygmomanometer on the pressure infusor is maintained higher than the patient's systolic blood pressure, the drip is easily maintained. Blood for blood gas determinations may be drawn from the arterial catheter. The line needs to be flushed thoroughly with the heparinized solution after any blood samples are withdrawn. The calibration of the machine needs to be rechecked at least once every eight hours.

Central Venous Pressure

Venous pressure arises from the arterial pressure transmitted across the capillary bed into the venous reservoir. A high venous pressure is often accompanied by full distended neck veins when the patient is in the semi-Fowler's position. The central venous pressure (CVP) (measured by a catheter in one of the main veins or in the right atrium) reflects the competency of the heart to handle the volume of blood being returned to it. It shows how the circulating blood volume compares with the pumping capacity of the heart at any particular time. It is of particular value in the bleeding patient as a guide to blood volume replacement when the hematocrit is inaccurate because of the latent period involved in the hemodilution process. A drop of

3 to 5 cm in water pressure may indicate that the patient has lost 10 percent of his blood volume [53]. The principal limitation of the CVP measurement is that it does not differentiate between hypervolemia and a failing heart; nor does it differentiate between hypovolemia and impeded venous return. Normal central venous pressure is between 5 and 15 cm H_2O, but the trend of the venous pressure and the response to therapy are often much more significant than the actual level of an isolated recording. The physician usually asks to be notified when the pressure changes abruptly, or is less than 5 or more than 15 cm H_2O.

The CVP catheter may be placed into the subclavian, superior vena cava, or right atrium from various external sites such as the median cubital, basilic, or cephalic vein of the arm. The jugular vein is occasionally used.

Although the CVP may be measured with a transducer in a manner similar to the central arterial pressure, it is more commonly measured with a water manometer by means of a three-way stopcock. The zero on the manometer must always be at the level of the right atrium. The right atrium is located inferiorly to midsternum and halfway from the front to the back of the chest. This is termed the reference position and should be marked with a felt pen so the zero on the manometer can be placed at this level for subsequent readings (Fig. 6–6). Using a carpenter's level and keeping the patient supine make the readings more accurate. If the patient is coughing, straining, or on the respirator, the reading may be abnormally high. The patient is not usually removed from the respirator for the readings, but this variable is taken into account when evaluating the reading.

Fluid must drip slowly into the system at all times except during the reading time. Medications are often added through the CVP line. Physicians are not in agreement about the advisability of adding drugs that have a stimulating effect on the heart muscle to the CVP line if the catheter is in the right atrium. Many physicians add any intravenous medication to a CVP line, but some prefer to give potassium chloride, aminophylline, and isoproterenol through another IV line.

Left Atrial Pressure

Left atrial pressure (LAP) is the direct reflection of the left ventricular end-diastolic pressure, or filling pressure. It reflects the cardiac output or the maximal capacity of the left ventricle to

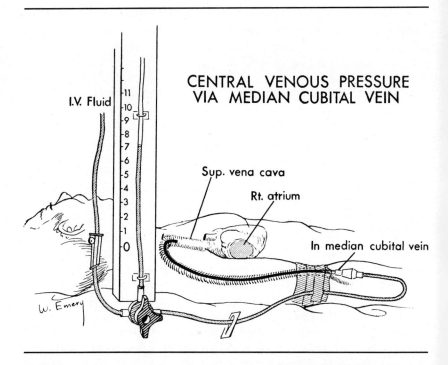

CENTRAL VENOUS PRESSURE
VIA MEDIAN CUBITAL VEIN

I.V. Fluid

Sup. vena cava

Rt. atrium

In median cubital vein

W. Emery

FIGURE 6–6   To measure the central venous pressure, the zero on the fluid-filled manometer is placed at the level of the right atrium and the stopcock is turned so that the intravenous line is open to the manometer. The fluid column in the manometer falls until it equals the pressure at the right atrial level. *(From D. Gilbo, Nursing Assessment of Circulatory Function, Nursing Clinics of North America, 3(1968). Used by permission of the author and W. B. Saunders Company, Philadelphia.)*

develop a volume load. It is the most reliable measurement for fluid replacement, since it gives earlier warning than the CVP of the development of heart failure.

The maintenance of adequate perfusion under conditions of impaired myocardial contractility is dependent upon deriving maximal left ventricular output, so some physicians deliberately maintain the left atrial pressure at abnormally high levels to increase the cardiac output [54]. Normal left atrial pressure is 8 to 18 cm H_2O. Usually it is 3 to 5 cm H_2O higher than the CVP, but the LAP cannot be predicted from the CVP. In cardiac postoperative patients, it may range from 12 to 25 cm H_2O; at 30 cm pulmonary edema usually develops, although it may develop at less than 30 cm.

In addition to the measurement of left atrial pressure, the left atrial catheter has been used for [54]:

1   Measurement of cardiac output by direct infusion of indicator dye into the left atrium

2   Visualization of a mitral valve prosthesis by the injection of a contrast medium

3   Securing a left atrial cardiogram when the P waves could not be visualized with the standard placement of leads

To measure the LAP, a small polyethylene catheter must be inserted into the left atrium at the time of surgery before the thoracotomy wound is closed. The catheter is brought out through the chest wall and secured with a suture. The LAP is usually measured with a water manometer in the same manner as the central venous pressure. A heparinized solution should run at a slow drip except during the periods a reading is being taken. No drugs except heparin should be added to the LAP line. Precautions must be taken to prevent air or clots entering the system, since 0.1 ml of air has been found to cause myocardial ischemia in animals [55]. Since any patient with multiple lines and IV flush bottles is susceptible to errors in addition of fluids and medications to lines due to lines becoming entwined, each line should be labeled appropriately just below the drip chamber and also at the tape securing the insertion of the needle or catheter.

Heart Rate and Sounds

Heart rate and sounds give an indication of the character of the heart's contraction. Patients with prosthetic ball valves have a sound that accompanies the closing of the valve. A developing murmur is usually an indication of malfunction.

Temperature of the Great Toe

Temperature of the great toe, measured with a thermistor probe, is sometimes monitored since a high correlation has been found between the cardiac output and the toe temperature [56].

Peripheral Circulation

An indication of the adequacy of *tissue perfusion* is given by the temperature, color, and fullness of veins of the extremities and the presence and strength of radial, femoral, carotid, popliteal, dorsalis pedis, and posterior tibial pulses (Fig. 6–7). In order to make recording of pulses and skin perfusion more uniform, the following scale can be used:

4+ Strong pedal and radial pulses. Skin warm and pink. Veins full.

3+ Pedal and radial pulses palpable. Extremities pale and cool. Slow venous filling.

2+ Strong central pulses. Peripheral pulses questionable. Moderate cyanosis of lips and nailbeds. Extremities cool.

1+ Weak femoral and carotid pulses only. Extremities cold. Deeply cyanotic.

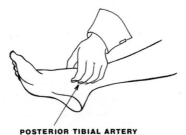

POSTERIOR TIBIAL ARTERY

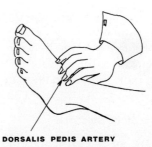

DORSALIS PEDIS ARTERY

PERIPHERAL PULSES

FIGURE 6–7 With practice, the nurse can become skillful in estimating the cardiac output from the temperature, color, and character of the pulses in the feet.

When the cardiac output is less than 2 l/min, the perfusion index will probably only be 1+ or 2+.

Renal Perfusion

Many factors can interfere with renal function, but if the urinary output is 30 cc or more per hour, the kidney is usually being adequately perfused.

Cerebral Perfusion

Inadequate circulation to the brain usually results in a lowered level of cerebral functioning. Indicators of cerebral circulation are (1) sensorium—alert or obtunded, (2) pupil size and reaction to light, and (3) strength of handgrips.

Psychological Response

Impairment of normal physiological function and/or emotional reaction to the surgical procedure often result in psychological disturbances. The normal individual has a mature and integrated cognitive system with which he organizes and manipulates the world around him. He can use the past to help him understand the present and to plan constructively and realistically for the future. Some manifestations of cognitive or psychological disturbances are inability to interpret adequately the environment, and disturbed behavior. These disturbances will be discussed more fully in the section under stress.

Impulse Formation and Conduction

The electrocardiogram is a graphic tracing that shows three aspects of the heart's electrical activity: timing, magnitude, and direction. The electrocardiograph paper is divided into squares by a series of lines that measure time horizontally and a series of lines that measure voltage vertically.

Measurement of Time

Each side of a large square on the electrocardiograph paper is 5 mm in length. Each large square is divided into small squares 1 mm in length. Since the paper usually moves through the machine at a rate of 25 mm/sec, five large squares are used to record 1 sec. Three hundred large squares equal 1 min. Each large square represents 0.20 sec, and each small square represents 0.04 sec (Fig. 6–8).

Measurement of Voltage

Voltage magnitude is indicated by the vertical displacement of the stylus. A 10-mm displacement represents 1 mv of electromotive force.

Measurement of Direction

The direction of the electrical depolarization of the heart muscle has been termed the electrical axis. Normal depolarization progresses from the endocardium to the outside surfaces of the ventricles. Since the left ventricle is the largest muscle body, the left ventricular forces are the largest, causing the axis to point to the left and downward. The normal range of axes on the hexaxial scale is −30° to +120° [52].

Components of the EKG

Einthoven arbitrarily designated the forces as the P wave, QRS complex, T wave, and U wave. The U wave is a low-voltage wave and

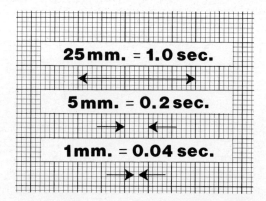

REPRESENTATION OF TIME
ON EKG PAPER

FIGURE 6–8   Arrows indicate the length of the EKG paper that corresponds to each time.

sometimes is not seen. The various waveforms of the electrocardiogram represent differing electrical events occurring in the myocardium. The P wave represents the activation and the depolarization of the atria (the sinus impulse is not seen on the electrocardiograph). The PR segment is the spread of the impulse through the AV node to the ventricles. The QRS complex indicates the depolarization of the ventricles. The ST segment is the period of rest between depolarization and repolarization of the ventricles, with the T wave representing the repolarization of the ventricles. Repolarization of the atria is obscured on the electrocardiogram by the QRS complex (Fig. 6–9).

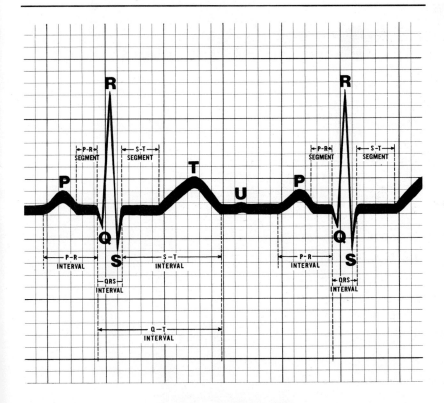

EKG COMPLEX

FIGURE 6–9   A diagramatic representation of the electrocardiogram with identification of the various components, intervals, and segments.

The PR interval, which is the period from the start of the P wave to the beginning of the QRS complex, should be between 0.1 and 0.21 sec.

The QRS complex consists of an initial downward deflection (Q wave), a large upward deflection (R wave), and a second downward wave (S wave). The Q and the S waves may be absent, but it is still referred to as the QRS complex. The normal duration of this impulse is less than 0.12 sec.

The heart *rate* can be computed quickly from an EKG strip by counting the number of large squares between the R waves and dividing 300 by that number. For greater accuracy, interpolation can be made for fractions of squares. Another method of calculating the heart rate is to count the number of R waves in a 6-in. strip of the electrocardiographic paper. Since 6 in. is equivalent to 6 sec, the number of R waves can be multiplied by 10 to get the rate. EKG paper is marked at the top margin in 3-in. intervals, so this is an easy method.

Approach to Studying an EKG

Although monitor leads cannot be used for definitive diagnosis, a systematic approach should be used in the study of any EKG. The usual factors identified are:

1 Type of rhythm (regular or irregular)

2 Determination of rate

3 Presence or absence of P wave

4 Measurement of PR interval duration

5 Measurement of duration of QRS complex

6 Configuration of QRS complex

7 Elevation or depression of the ST segment

8 Direction, shape, and height of the T wave

9 Presence of the U wave

Technical Aspects of the EKG Tracing

In order to reduce the variables that influence or distort the EKG, the nurse who is monitoring a patient's EKG needs to use a careful technique. *Standardization* should be carefully checked. The EKG standardization is 1 mv, which should result in a 10-mm deflection of the baseline (two large squares).

Good electrical contact is essential to avoid artifacts. The electrode jelly should be rubbed briskly on the skin and the electrode should fit snugly.

Patient position should be uniform, preferably with the patient flat when any strips are taken for the record. *Identification of the lead used* should be made on any strip placed in the record, if the monitoring machine is one that allows selection of lead.

Placement of the electrode should be accurate. Although monitoring leads cannot be used alone for diagnosis of abnormal heart rhythms, they can provide a record of change and are more reliable when they are consistently placed. When disks on the chests are used for monitoring instead of electrodes on the extremities, they are frequently placed to simulate Lead II. In such cases, the proper placement is (Fig. 6–10):

Positive lead (black in standard sets) on the left upper chest near the shoulder.

Negative lead (white in standard sets) on the right upper chest near the shoulder.

Ground lead (red in standard sets) on the left side below the diaphragm. Monitor should be set on Lead II.

A new method, the *Modified Chest Lead* I (MCL₁), has been suggested by Dr. Henry J. L. Marriott and adopted by many intensive care units [57]. This lead simulates V₁ position (fourth interspace at the right sternal edge). It allows flexibility since one can relocate the positive electrode to the V₆ position (MCL₆) or the left leg position to provide a modified Lead III (M₃). When monitoring MCL₁, the monitor should be set on Lead I and the proper placement of the leads is (Fig. 6–11): positive lead on the fourth intercostal space just to the right of the sternum; negative lead just below the outer third of the left clavicle. Ground can be placed anywhere, but is usually just below the right clavicle.

Alternate placements to MCL₁ are: for MCL₆, the positive electrode is on the midaxillary line at the level of the fifth intercostal space; for M₃, the positive electrode is on the left abdomen below the diaphragm.

The diagnostic advantages of the MCL₁ are:

Can switch easily to MCL₆ or M₃.

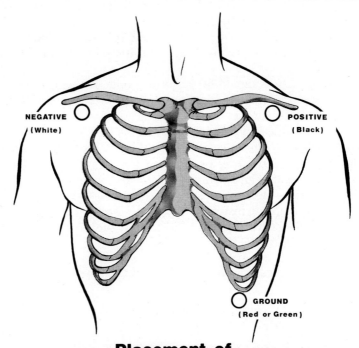

NEGATIVE ○ (White)

POSITIVE ○ (Black)

○ GROUND (Red or Green)

Placement of
MONITORING ELECTRODES
FOR SIMULATED LEAD II

FIGURE 6–10

Can distinguish between left ventricular ectopy and aberrant conduction of the right bundle-branch block (RBBB) type.

Left ventricular ectopy has a qR in MCL₁ and an rS in MCL₆. RBBB-type aberration gives a triphasic rSR′ in the MCL₁ and a qRs in MCL₆.

Can determine if ventricular ectopies such as extrasystoles, spontaneous rhythms, or pacemaker rhythms are from the right or left ventricle. Ventricular extrasystoles from the left ventricle are more likely to trigger ventricular fibrillation [57].

Left ventricular ectopy has a qR in MCL₁ (positive deflection). Right ventricular ectopy has an rS in MCL₁ (negative deflection).

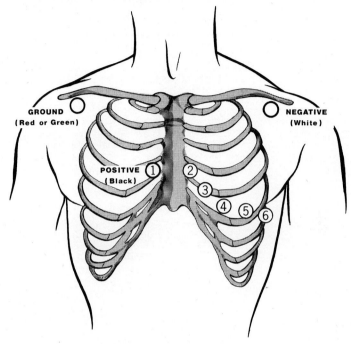

GROUND
(Red or Green)

NEGATIVE
(White)

POSITIVE
(Black)

Placement of

MONITORING ELECTRODES FOR M C L$_1$

FIGURE 6–11

Can distinguish between RBBB and LBBB.

RBBB has an rSR' in MCL$_1$ and a qRs in MCL$_6$.
LBBB has an rS in MCL$_1$ and a monophasic positive R wave in MCL$_6$.

Can identify the presence of retrograde polarity of the P waves in AV junctional rhythms by the use of M$_3$.

Abnormal Heart Rhythms

The term *arrhythmia* is often used in reference to abnormal patterns of heart conduction, but this term is inaccurate and is being replaced by the more descriptive term "abnormal heart rhythms." Some of the more commonly occurring abnormal heart rates and/or rhythms are shown in the following table:

Condition	Type of Rhythm
Tachycardia	Fast, regular. May originate in the atria, AV node, or the ventricle. Sinus tachycardia is a rate in excess of 100 min.
Bradycardia	Slow, regular. Sinus bradycardia has a rate slower than 60/min.
Flutter	Very fast, regular, characterized by sawtooth undulations of the baseline. May originate in either the atria or the ventricles.
Fibrillation	Fast but extremely irregular, with bizarre abnormalities of the electrocardiogram's wave structure. May originate in either the atria or the ventricles.
Arrest	Has intervals of time during which the heart does not beat.
Block	Characterized by a delay or interruption in the depolarization pathway of the heart. May occur in the SA node, AV node, or the branches of the bundle of His.
Wenckebach	Type of 2d degree block of the AV node in which there is a progressive increase in the P-R interval with a decrease in the R-R interval until there is a dropped beat.
Premature contractions or extrasystoles	Isolated occurrences that interrupt the prevailing heart rhythm. May be caused by an ectopic force in the atria, AV node, or the ventricles.
Multifocal ectopic beats	Premature beats arising from more than one focus.
Bigeminy	Premature extrasystoles that are coupled or alternated with a sinus contraction. Ectopic beat may come from the atria (atrial bigeminy) or the ventricle (ventricular bigeminy).
Interpolated beat	Extremely premature beat sandwiched between two consecutive sinus beats. Since the ectopic beat occurs so early, the ventricle has sufficient time to recover and is thus able to respond.
Parasystole	Autonomous ectopic focus that fires at an independent rate. If an impulse arises outside of the refractory period, an ectopic beat that has a variable coupling relationship to the sinus beats will be produced.
Fusion beats	Combination of a sinus and an ectopic impulse that occurs when the two impulses enter the ventricular myocardium at the same time, producing a QRS-T complex that is intermediate in form between the sinus and ectopic beats.
Idioventricular rhythm	Originating in an ectopic ventricular pacemaker.
Ventricular aberration	Temporary abnormal intraventricular conduction of a supraventricular impulse. It is important to distinguish it from ventricular ectopy, since the treatment of the two differs greatly.

Condition	Type of Rhythm
Wandering pacemaker	Alteration in the configuration of the P wave because the pacemaker moves from the SA node to other locations in the atria.
AV or junctional rhythms (sometimes called nodal rhythms)	Originating in the AV node.
AV dissociation	Atria and ventricle beating independently of each other. May result from a block of the AV node or from an accelerated ventricular pacemaker that takes over the pacing of the heart. If atrial and ventricular rates are nearly identical, it is termed isorhythmic dissociation or accrochage.
Escape beat	Ectopic beat that ends a longer than usual cycle of the dominant pacer.

Patients who have heart surgery with cardiopulmonary bypass may have varied and complex abnormal heart rhythms. The abnormal rhythms may be caused by intracardiac surgical manipulation, trauma of the SA node from cannulation of the vena cava, damage to the AV node from suction in the coronary sinus, or underlying heart defects. Many factors may contribute to the abnormal rhythms, including hypoxemia, ischemia, potassium level, acid-base imbalance, myocardial failure, and certain drugs. It is rather common for highly skilled cardiologists to disagree on whether a particular abnormality is caused by aberrant conduction or ventricular ectopy. The surgical nurse needs to have a greater knowledge of abnormal EKG rhythms than is usually received in a short course or discussion of the common

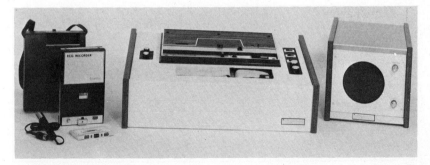

FIGURE 6–12   The portable EKG recorder (left) in its carrying case with shoulder or belt strap monitors the heart as the patient goes about his normal activities. The 8-hr casette allows voice recording simulaneously with the EKG. The playback equipment consists of a reproduction system (center) and an oscilloscope display (right). The tape can be viewed in real time or in the scan mode, which allows 8 hr of data to be viewed in 15 min. *(Photograph courtesy of Intermed Corporation, Dallas, Texas.)*

disorders of the heart. For that reason, this manual needs to be supplemented by a textbook on electrocardiography, or by an in-depth course in EKG interpretation.

The monitor strips of the EKG activity are usually attached to the nursing notes every 2 hr for the first 48 hr after surgery and then at

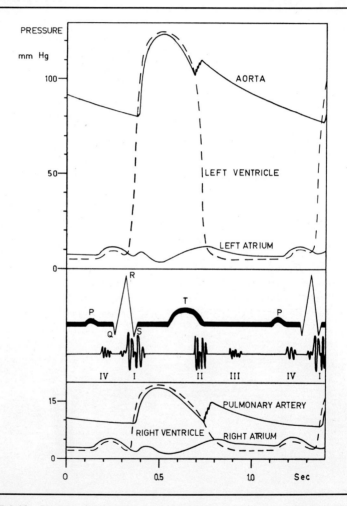

FIGURE 6–13 Diagram of the relationships of the various electrical and mechanical events in the cardiac cycle. From the bottom to the top, the events depicted are the right atrial pressure, right ventricular pressure, pulmonary artery pressure, heart sounds, electrocardiogram, left atrial pressure, left ventricular pressure, and central arterial (aortic) pressure. *(From Alan C. Burton, "Physiology and Biophysics of the Circulation," Year Book Medical Publishers, Inc., Chicago, 1965. Used by permission.)*

8-hr intervals. A strip of any change in pattern should always be placed on the record. If the leads are changed from the previous strip, this information should be included.

Some patients have more abnormal heart rhythms with activity than they have at rest. For these patients, portable EKG readings may be obtained by the use of a medical data recorder (Fig. 6–12). Sample EKG strips with accompanying interpretations are listed in Appendix E. Assessment is never based on a single parameter, but on a composite of observations and measurements. An understanding of the interrelationships between the BP, LAP, and the electrical and mechanical events of the cardiac cycle is crucial (Fig. 6–13).

NURSING MEASURES TO PROMOTE ADEQUATE CIRCULATION IN THE POSTOPERATIVE PERIOD

Measures	Rationale
Elevate the entire head of bed at least 30 °.	Gravity pressure on the lower extremities must be maintained or the part of the total blood volume usually distributed to the legs is redistributed to other parts of the body, increasing the volume of circulating blood that must be handled by the heart [58].
Encourage and assist with range of motion exercises every 1 to 2 hr starting with patient's arrival from operating room.	Muscular pressure on veins is needed to assist return flow of blood to the heart.
Especially include dorsiflexion and hyperextension of the feet, and flattening of the knee to the mattress.	Stretching the muscles in the calves of the legs helps prevent formation of a thrombus because of venous stasis.
Keep knees flat without using knee gatch or pillow when patient is on his back, and position his legs so one leg does not rest heavily on the other when he is on his side.	External pressure on blood vessels of legs, especially pressure on the popliteal space where vessels are superficial and easily injured, results in a layer of platelets being laid down over the injured blood vessel intima that may form the basis for a blood clot.
Wrap the legs with elastic bandages from toes to above knees, or apply antiembolic stocking. Remove for a short period every 6 to 8 hr.	Firm pressure on legs helps prevent venous stasis.

NURSING MEASURES TO PROMOTE ADEQUATE CIRCULATION IN THE POSTOPERATIVE
PERIOD *(Continued)*

Measures	Rationale
Turn patient every 2 hr, instructing him to exhale as he is turned.	Pressure exerted against the closed glottis with breath-holding and the resultant thorax fixation elevates the intrathoracic pressure which in turn decreases the venous gradient and interferes with entry of venous blood into large veins. When the breath is then released, intrathoracic pressure drops and a large surge of blood is delivered to the heart at one time which may overburden the heart. The rush of blood may also produce enough force to loosen a fragile, slightly detached blood clot from the lower extremity. The phenomenon of thoracic fixation without expiration has been termed a Valsalva maneuver if the intrathoracic pressure is elevated above 40 mm Hg for a period of 8 sec [59].
Encourage use of a bedside commode that allows the patient's feet to rest flat on floor. Give stool softeners as ordered to make straining unnecessary.	Straining at stool can initiate the Valsalva maneuver. Use of the bedpan for stool increases the normal strain by 50 percent [59].
Keep anxiety from becoming too severe.	Anxiety results in increased secretion of catecholamines and may have a deleterious effect on the heart's action.
Use a special boot (such as the Spenco boot by Stryker) during surgery and a foot board after surgery.	Peroneal nerve damage that may result in foot drop can occur when foot is not properly supported.
Keep arterial catheter taped securely and area immobilized. Inspect frequently for any area of anesthesia or impairment of function.	Nerves are easily damaged by needles in adjacent arteries.
Administer medication as ordered for abnormal heart rhythms, for blood pressure abnormalities, or for severe peripheral arterial constriction.	Irregularities in heart rhythm may lead to serious cardiac problems if not promptly treated. A drop in blood pressure may indicate a lowered cardiac output inadequate to meet the demands of the body. A high rise in blood pressure may lead to rupture of a blood vessel graft and/or suture line. Severe arterial constriction interferes with maintenance of tissue life.

NURSING MEASURES TO PROMOTE ADEQUATE CIRCULATION IN THE POSTOPERATIVE
PERIOD *(Continued)*

Measures	Rationale
Maintain temperature within normal range (or at least under 101°) by the use of acetylsalicylic acid suppositories, alcohol and warm water sponges, or hypothermia blanket as ordered by the doctor.	Elevation of temperature increases the metabolic requirement for oxygen and places a greater strain upon the heart. The metabolic rate increases 13 percent for each 1°C and 8 percent for each 1°F [60]. Sponging results in heat loss by evaporation, thus a warm mixture of water and alcohol cools almost as effectively as an ice-cold solution, with less discomfort.
Give careful attention to skin care, especially if tissue is edematous or bones are prominent. Use air mattress or sheepskin where indicated.	Skin breakdown is a frequent problem when there is impairment of circulation or areas of increased pressure.
If bed rest will be prolonged, transfer patient to a Circ-Olectric bed and position him nearly upright with weight-bearing on his feet several times a day.	Weight-bearing on the feet promotes venous return. The upright position maintains efficiency of the orthostatic neurovascular reflex control of blood vessels so that patient does not experience orthostatic hypotension.
Maintain as quiet an environment as possible and space nursing activities to provide for periods of maximum rest.	Periods of rest are necessary to promote restoration and repair of cells of body. Tissue needs for oxygen are decreased when body is at a resting state.
When oral feeding is permitted, give diet in six small, equal portions.	Blood is shunted to the splanchnic-mesenteric arteries for metabolism and absorption of food, lowering the blood supply to the heart and other vital organs. Large meals put pressure on the diaphragm and may cause respiratory problems.

SHOCK

7

Shock may be defined as a clinical state of inadequate tissue perfusion that results from a decreased effective circulating blood volume. In early shock, homeostatic processes cause sympathetic stimulation with an increased secretion of norepinephrine, which results in peripheral vasoconstriction and diversion of blood from nonvital peripheral areas in order to maintain adequate tissue perfusion of vital organs. As time passes, if the underlying cause is not corrected, the lack of cellular oxygen in the microcirculation retards the normal process of metabolic oxidation and anaerobic metabolism results in lactic acid accumulating in the tissue fluid, which eventually leads to metabolic acidosis. With increased acidosis, the arteriolar sphincters lose their tone and the arteries become dilated, and the veins remain constricted. Thus blood is pooled and trapped in the peripheral circulatory system. Shock is sometimes termed *stagnant* or *irreversible* when the blood or blood volume expanders given are retained in the active circulation for only a short period of time before they are forced out into the tissues. If the systolic blood pressure is less than 60 for four hours or more, irreversible damage to the reticular system will probably result as cellular hypoxia progresses to tissue asphyxia.

CLASSIFICATION

Although all types of shock result in cellular hypoxia, the hemo-dynamic alterations and the underlying problem responsible for the condition need to be identified for therapy to be effective. Shock has been classified into various subgroups depending on the etiology. One of the most popular methods utilizes the following three categories:

- *Cardiogenic.* Caused by cardiac pump failure
- *Hematogenic* or *hypovolemic.* Caused by a decrease in the volume of blood or fluid
- *Vasogenic.* Secondary to the dilatation of the blood vessels by toxic substances as bacteria (gram-negative shock) or histamine (anaphylactic shock)

Some cases of shock are caused by combinations of the above categories, and hypovolemic shock leads to the development of associated cardiogenic shock.

NURSING ASSESSMENT

Early symptoms of shock result from:

- Inability to adapt the circulation to the brain with changes in position
- Initiation of protective mechanisms as vasoconstriction, which may mask a considerable fall in cardiac output before hypotension is manifest
- Signs of increased sympathetic activity, which is the body's mechanism to control the shock

Although not all symptoms are characteristic of all categories of shock, the variables in the following table should be carefully assessed and recorded:

Variable	Manifestation
Skin	Cold, clammy, and mottled with cyanosis of the nailbeds except in septic shock. (Skin may be initially warm and dry in septic shock.)
State of consciousness	Anxiety, restlessness, and agitation, which may progress to confusion and ultimately coma.
Blood pressure	Drop in systolic blood pressure with a lesser reduction in diastolic pressure (thus narrow pulse pressure).

Variable	Manifestation
Central pulses	Rapid, weak, and thready.
Peripheral pulses	Diminished or absent.
Respiration	Rapid and shallow.
Urine output	Reduced, or may cease altogether.
Peripheral and neck veins	Collapsed, except in cardiogenic shock, in which case they may be distended.
Temperature (rectal)	May be elevated in septic shock.
Temperature measured by a thermistor taped to the great toe	When below 27°C, shock severe. When below 35°C but above 29.2°C, shock is moderate, with good prospect for recovery [56].
Metabolic state	Acidosis

PRINCIPLES OF TREATMENT

The treatment of shock is directed toward correcting, altering, or eliminating the basic underlying pathology while restoring the balance between the cardiac output and the peripheral flow.

Eight years of study at the Shock Research Unit of the University of Southern California has caused many physicians to question some of their formerly held assumptions and therapeutic measures for shock [61]. Some of their findings are:

- Respiratory failure is the single most frequent cause of death. Thus the Trendelenburg position, which increases the work of breathing, is no longer recommended for the patient in shock.

- Keeping the body warm produces vasodilation, which may further decrease the already impaired volume of circulating blood. Therefore, no blankets are used on the patient in shock.

- The use of vasopressor drugs is sometimes more detrimental than beneficial, particularly when the blood volume is markedly depleted, so their use in shock is usually limited.

The therapeutic approach proposed by the Shock Research Unit to replace the former methods of management has been termed the "VIP" approach, which stands for ventilate, infuse, and pump. These actions are then followed by pharmacological and/or surgical management based on the VIP diagnostic data. Advocates of this approach feel it gives them a priority sequence for a series of therapeutic-diagnostic measures that will control, or at least delay, the most immediate threat while providing the diagnostic information needed to proceed rationally to the next step [61]. The rationale for the VIP approach in brief is:

- *Ventilate* to maintain a normal PO_2 that will help to minimize ischemic injuries to the vital organs and tissues. Respirators are usually used. The adequacy of pulmonary ventilation is assessed by measurement of the arterial oxygen tension.

- *Infuse* to restore blood, fluid, electrolyte, and acid-base balance, using the central venous pressure as a volume guide, and to provide diagnostic information. To differentiate between cardiogenic and hypovolemic shock, the fluid challenge response is obtained by giving 200 cc of saline in 10 min. A rise in CVP in excess of 5 cm H_2O (without an increase in BP) indicates limited cardiac competence. A rise in BP without a significant change in the CVP indicates that hypovolemia is probably present. The cardio-vascular response to the challenge of a fluid load has been said to be the single most important measurement that can be made in the shock patient [12].

- *Pump* deficiencies should be corrected to improve cardiac competence. Main methods to improve the output are the administration of digitalis and the correction of any arrhythmias that impair cardiac output. In some instances, a phlebotomy may be indicated.

After the data obtained from the VIP approach have been correlated with the other findings and symptoms, additional therapy that is specific for each category of shock should be instituted. All medications should be given intravenously since intramuscular medications are poorly absorbed when the peripheral circulation is decreased.

Cardiogenic Shock

Cardiogenic shock is a rather frequent development after open-heart surgery, especially surgery for aortic valvular disease [38]. A patient who has a cardiac output of less than 2 l/min/sq m of body surface is said to have the "low-output syndrome" [54]. Hypovolemia may be a contributing cause to low-output syndrome. Some causes of impairment of the myocardial function are:

- Myocardial ischemia, which may be caused by coronary air embolus during operation or interrupted coronary artery perfusion
- Arrhythmias associated with an inadequate stroke volume

- Cross clamping of aorta for more than 30 min
- Myocardial depression by anesthetics and hypothermia
- Trauma of operation
- Mechanical impedance to contraction caused by implanted prosthetic valve
- Decreased compliance of the ventricle because of scar tissue or hypertrophy
- Decreased contractility of muscle fibers that results from the long period of bypass inactivity
- Preexisting heart disease not corrected by surgery

Therapy

Therapy for cardiogenic shock is directed toward the improvement of myocardial contractility. Some aspects are:

Vasoconstrictors

Most surgeons avoid the use of vasoconstrictive drugs since increasing the central arterial pressure increases the cardiac work without necessarily improving the blood flow. Furthermore, most of these patients have strong central pulses with severe peripheral vasoconstriction and resultant metabolic acidosis, which makes the heart muscle function less effectively.

Isuprel

Isuprel is the preferred catecholamine of most surgeons. It has an inotropic as well as a chronotropic effect on the heart. It has a dilator effect on the peripheral blood vessels and decreases the peripheral and pulmonary vascular resistance. Thus it improves the cardiac function and reduces the resistance against which the heart must pump. Also, by decreasing the volume capacity of the venous system, it increases the venous return. The administration needs to be carefully monitored since sometimes in large doses the action is reversed. An electronic infusion pump such as the Ivac 500 provides a safe method of administration. Undesirable side effects of Isuprel are tachycardia; ventricular irritability with extrasystoles and possible ventricular fibrillation; and inspissation of bronchial secretions.

Alpha-adrenergic blockers

These cause vasodilatation and are recommended by some surgeons for cardiogenic shock with severe peripheral vasoconstriction. Phenoxybenzamine (Dibenzyline) and phenotolamine (Regitine) have both been used successfully to improve tissue perfusion, increase cardiac output, and decrease venous pressure [12]. Surgeons at St. Vincent's Hospital in Los Angeles give small bolus doses of chlorpromazine (Thorazine), 4 to 16 mg intravenously every 1 to 2 hr; other surgeons advocate the intravenous administration of a dilute solution of trimetaphan camphorsulfonate (Arfonad) [38].

If the blood pressure is below 50, some surgeons use a combination of a vasopressor with an adrenergic blocking drug such as phenoxybenzamine (Dibenzyline) or phentolamine (Regitine). The drugs block the alpha-adrenergic receptors in the wall of the blood vessels, so the vasoconstrictor effect of the catecholamine is abolished but the inotropic effect on the heart is preserved [12].

Digitalis

Digitalis significantly increases the strength of contraction in the failing heart. Experimental work has also shown that digitalis can increase the degree of oxygen debt that can be tolerated [12]. Intravenous preparations of deslanoside (Cedilanid) are usually given slowly for digitalization. Ouabain may be given for faster action, but its period of activity is short. When fresh blood is not available for transfusion and bank blood is used, the high-potassium, high-acid, and low-sodium concentrations adversely affect the digitalization process.

Morphine Sulfate

Three to five mg intravenously usually improves cardiogenic shock.

Antiacidosis Drugs

These drugs are usually given to combat the progressive metabolic acidosis that decreases the force of the heart muscle contraction and may lead to ventricular fibrillation. The vasomotor system is unresponsive to catecholamines when the pH of the blood falls below 7. The effectiveness of alkali therapy when hypercapnia is present has been questioned by some physicians who advocate intensive pulmonary care for metabolic acidosis accompanied by respiratory acidosis, and individualization of the amount of alkali used based on blood studies rather than routinely giving large amounts of buffers [62].

Sodium bicarbonate, given for metabolic acidosis with a pH below 7, is usually not given faster than 3 mEq/min [12]. It is available as a 7.5 percent solution in a 50-cc ampule that contains 44.6 mEq. It is also available as a 5 percent solution in a 500-cc intravenous bottle that contains 44.6 mEq in each 75 cc.

Trihydroxy aminomethane (THAM) is a powerful hydrogen-ion acceptor that seems to be effective for respiratory acidosis as well as metabolic acidosis since it combines with CO_2. It also has the ability to cross the cell membrane and counteract intracellular acidosis [12]. Precautions that should be used in the administration of THAM are:

1 THAM needs to be diluted in fairly large volumes of fluid because of its alkalinity (pH 12). Eighteen grams of THAM are diluted with 500 cc fluid to give a 0.3 molar solution.

2 It should not be given unless the patient is on a respirator or a respirator is readily available because it is a powerful respiratory depressant.

3 Frequent monitoring of the pH is necessary to detect developing alkalosis.

Adrenocorticosteroids

Adrenocorticosteriods are sometimes given, although their efficacy in cardiogenic shock is equivocable. Large doses are needed to get an inotropic effect.

Glucagon

Glucagon has been advocated by some physicians as a means of increasing cardiac output [63]. A hormone secreted by the pancreas, glucagon increases the blood glucose level by speeding the conversion of glycogen to glucose, but it also has a positive inotropic and chronotropic effect on the heart. It increases the heart rate, stroke volume, cardiac output, and arterial pressure. The effect is transient, with the maximum effect within 7 to 10 min, and dissipation of effectiveness after 15 to 20 min. Generally 5 to 10 mg is given intravenously every 15 min. There has not been adequate testing for its continued use over a long period of time, and its value is controversial.

Mechanical Cardiac Assistance

This is sometimes given temporarily with counterpulsion devices and intraaortic balloon pumps (sometimes termed diastolic pumps), although their use is still mainly in the experimental stage [13].

Paired Pulsations

Paired pulsations by a pacing electrode have been used experimentally to treat intractable tachycardias and augment myocardial contractility. This method takes advantage of the potentiation of an impulse that follows the compensatory pause after a premature contraction. When paired pulses are delivered to the myocardium by a pacing electrode, only every other beat is transmitted The contraction that then results is augmented with a greater volume of output caused by increased diastolic filling [29].

Hematogenic or Hypovolemic Shock

Hematogenic shock is a common complication of open-heart surgery. The average blood volume is about 5 liters in an adult. Studies have shown that in the normal patient the loss of 500 ml of blood can be tolerated with no drop in cardiac output. Mild shock is usually associated with a blood loss of 15 to 20 percent (1000 ml in adult), moderate shock with 20 to 35 percent and severe shock with a blood loss that approaches 50 percent of the volume [29]. Not only is the total blood volume significant, but the proportion of the red blood cells to the fluid or plasma is important. This proportion is expressed as the *hematocrit*. The normal hematocrit is 45 for a man and 40 for a woman. This means that 45 percent of the blood volume of a man is composed of red blood cells.

Sometimes the amount of *hemoglobin* is measured instead of the proportion of red blood cells. Normally blood has approximately 15 gm of hemoglobin per 100 ml of blood. After a massive loss of blood, the hematocrit or hemoglobin value may not drop immediately. However, hemodilution takes place as fluid is given and blood loss is not replaced by blood and both the hematocrit and hemoglobin value will drop. A drop in hemoglobin of 1 gm or hematocrit of 2 percent usually indicates a loss of one unit (500 ml) of blood. Some causes of hypovolemia are:

- *Inadequate volume* of fluid and blood replaced during surgical period.

- *Vasodilatation* from rewarming after surgery.

- *Extensive fluid shifts* and sequestration of blood and extra-cellular fluid in the body cavities and in the interstitial spaces.

- *Hemorrhage,* which, in the usual order of frequency of occurrence may be caused by:

  Fibrinolysis, in which fibrinogen is being converted into fibrin so a clot is formed but some abnormal system within the body is producing fibrinolysin, which causes the clot to be absorbed or destroyed. Fibrinolysin is produced by the body during bypass so prolonged periods of cardiopulmonary bypass (more than 2½ hr) as well as platelet deficiency following bypass will increase fibrinolysis. Patients who had cyanotic heart disease and developed a compensatory polycythemia and those with poor liver function caused by congestive failure also have increased fibrinolysis. Sometimes euglobulin analysis assay is used to evaluate fibrinolytic activity. A lysis time of less than 45 min is usually associated with increased bleeding [64]. A simpler test that may be done at the bedside is to allow a 5-ml sample of blood to clot in a test tube and stand for 30 min. Gentle shaking of the test tube should not break a normal clot, but will result in lysis of a clot when fibrinolytic activity is increased.

  Inadequate neutralization of heparin. Usually 300 units per kilogram of heparin are given to avoid clotting of blood while the patient is on the pump. Protamine sulfate is then given to counteract the effect of heparin, with 1.5 mg of protamine given for each 100 units of heparin. Protamine titrations can be done to determine if the patient needs more protamine.

  Active bleeder in the chest. Chest drainage optimally should be no more than 50 cc per hr. If the volume of blood draining from the chest continues to be more than 100 cc per hr eight hours after surgery and no other cause for the bleeding has been identified, the patient is usually reexplored. If the blood pressure drops below 70 systolic in surgery, bleeding will usually cease and thus the location of the bleeder may not be found.

  Clotting abnormalities. Although there are 12 factors responsible for blood clotting, an inadequate amount of any factor except fibrinogen is very rare.

The specific assessment of hypovolemia, in addition to the symptoms given, for all types of shock includes:

- Determination of the circulating blood volume by dye dilution techniques, which may be inaccurate for patients in shock

- Accurate, frequent measurement of blood in chest drainage bottles and maintenance of an hourly balance of the blood replaced in relationship to that lost
- Sunken eyes and loss of skin turgor
- Rise of systolic blood pressure without a significant rise in the central venous pressure when buffered isotonic saline is administered rapidly by the intravenous route

Therapy

Therapy for hypovolemic shock is directed toward replacing the volume deficit and treating the underlying cause, which includes surgical intervention for a bleeder, adequate neutralization of heparin, and control of fibrinolysis. Elevation of the legs without lowering of the head may be advisable since the resultant emptying of the leg veins is equivalent to a 500-ml transfusion.

Fluid Volume Replacement

A combination of blood, plasma, and an electrolyte solution like Ringer's lactate is usually used to replace the fluid volume. Since patients with advanced shock and acidosis cannot metabolize lactate readily, they may be treated with saline buffered with bicarbonate instead of lactate. Isotonic saline alone is rarely used without buffering since it has a pH around 5.5 and may contribute to the development of acidosis.

Since the oxygen-carrying capacity of the blood is nearly normal as long as the hematocrit is maintained above 30 percent, hemodilution is often desirable to reduce the heart's work and prevent red cell aggregation when the terminal blood vessels are constricted following shock [12]. Reexpansion of the extracellular space by replacing fluid that has shifted into the intracellular space, in addition to replacing fluid lost by frank hemorrhage, is essential to the successful combating of hypovolemic shock. It is sometimes advisable to give fluid until the patient has gained 2 or 3 kg of weight, as long as the CVP does not become elevated above 15 cm H_2O [12]. Serial chest x-rays every 2 to 4 hours will show enlargement of the heart and congestion of the lungs, which are indications that the rate of infusion needs to be slowed down and cardiotonic drugs given.

Plasma expanders, although not generally considered as effective as plasma, may be used when plasma is not available and it is mandatory to use molecules large enough to be retained in the vascular space. Clinical dextran (Dextran 75,000) and low molecular weight dextran (Dextran 40,000) are plasma expanders that rapidly expand the blood volume and may increase the cardiac output. In addition, low molecular weight dextran has been found to improve the micro-circulatory flow by preventing cell aggregation. However, its anti-coagulant effect may increase the bleeding so its use in hypovolemic shock is controversial.

Fresh blood (collected within 24 hr) is indicated whenever more than minimal hemorrhage is present because it contains the necessary clotting factors. Blood collected within 4 hr may be required if platelets are needed in addition to the plasma clotting factors. Packed red cells may be given instead of whole blood to a patient with congestive heart failure. Stored bank blood is undesirable, not only because it is low in calcium and other necessary clotting factors but also because it contains a high level of potassium that has been released from the blood cells during storage and which contributes to the development of acidosis.

Some guidelines for the administration of blood are:

- Blood should always be typed and completely crossmatched. When 24 hr has elapsed since previous transfusion, blood should be crossmatched with a newly drawn clot. The blood needs to be carefully checked with the patient to prevent error in adminis-tration. If incompatible blood is given, hemolysis of the donor cells by antibodies in the patient's plasma will result. Grossly incompatible blood may undergo rapid cell destruction with immediate (within 20 min) appearance of symptoms, but a slow rate of hemolysis may only be evidenced by the appearance of jaundice a few hours or days after the transfusion. Symptoms of a hemolytic transfusion reaction include feeling of warmth and tingling in the limb receiving infusion; constrictive pain in chest (sometimes bronchospasm); severe headache, lumbar pain, and leg pains; flushing of face, chills, and fever; tachypnea, tachycardia; hypotension and cyanosis; and jaundice, oliguria, and hemo-globinuria, which develop later.

- Other transfusion reactions should be watched for. Pyrogenic reactions usually result from the presence in the donor plasma of proteins to which the recipient is allergic, causing chills and hives. Pyogenic reactions, which are more severe, result from bacterial contamination. Both gram-negative and gram-positive contamina-tion can cause a pyogenic reaction, but a gram-negative reaction is usually more severe. Signs of a pyogenic reaction include elevation of temperature from 100 to 106°F, chills, backache, headache, general malaise, nausea, vomiting, and vascular collapse with hypotension. The transfusion should be stopped if signs of a pyogenic reaction occur.

- Every unit of blood should be checked for bilirubin content and discarded if elevated, to decrease the incidence of serum hepatitis. A more sophisticated test done in some hospitals is the testing for the hepatitis australian antigen by means of counterimmuno-electrophoresis.

- An inline blood microemboli filter (dacron wool) should be used for all blood administration.

- Blood should be warmed to near body temperature when it is given rapidly or it may cause hypothermia with an increase in metabolic acidosis and a decrease in cardiac output. A warming coil can be incorporated into the infusion line or the bag can be immersed in tepid water.

- More blood than is actually needed should never be given, as it has been found that the mortality rate is 75 percent in patients who receive more than 30 units of blood [65].

Control of Fibrinolysis and Other Clotting Abnormalities

Although fresh blood supplies the needed clotting factors for most patients, persistent bleeding may be an indication for the use of other agents. Such agents include:

1 *Platelet concentrate.* The volume of each unit of blood is reduced to 50 to 100 ml while retaining the platelets in a viable state. Usually 10 units of platelet concentrate are given at a time. They must be used soon after they are collected, so securing platelets is sometimes difficult. The red blood cells are returned to the donor, and the use of a closed system for withdrawal of blood, centrifugation, and reinfusion has increased the availability.

2 *Epsilon aminocaprolic acid* (Amicar or EACA), an antifibrinolysin former. The drug has no effect on fibrinolysin already formed. Initially 5 gm is usually given intravenously over a period of an hour, followed by a continuing infusion of 1 gm every hour for 8 to 10 hours. In some hospitals the administration of Amicar at the close of any major operation is routine; however, many authorities feel that it should be given only after test results

demonstrate a high level of fibrinolysis [66]. Amicar is contraindicated if the presence of an intravascular clot is suspected since it may permit massive propagation of the clot.

3 *Vitamin K* (AquaMephyton). Vitamin K may be given for the prothrombin deficiency that may result from the use of heparin or from inadequate synthesis of prothrombin from the liver. It is usually given intramuscularly, but 5 to 25 mg may be given intravenously at a rate that should never exceed 5 mg/min. Serial determinations of prothrombin time should be made whenever vitamin K is given.

4 *Protamine sulfate.* This drug is rarely given to control hemorrhage except in cases where there has been inadequate neutralization of heparin. An additional 20 to 50 mg given slowly intravenously over a period of 5 min is sometimes administered. A bedside test to determine the presence of the heparin factor may be made by adding 5 ml of blood from the patient to 5 ml of fresh unclotted control blood. Failure of the combined specimen to clot indicates the presence of heparin or heparin-like factor.

5 *Fibrinogen with antihemophilic factor* (Fibro-AHF). This is generally felt to be indicated when the serum fibrinogen is less than 100 mg per 100 ml of blood, or when the clotting time of the blood is more than 30 min. Since the incidence of viral hepatitis is higher than for any blood component [67], use of Fibro-AHF is usually reserved for patients who meet the criteria of low fibrinogen level listed above. It is also very expensive, costing approximately $150 a bottle. Two bottles (4 gm) are usually used initially, and most cases require 8 gm. Manufacturers' instructions for reconstitution and administration should be carefully followed. The manufacturers also outline a program of gamma globulin injection that they feel will help reduce the incidence of hepatitis.

6 *Heparin.* Heparin is given for disseminated intravascular coagulation in which the circulating plasma is changed to serum. The usual dose is one-third the calculated dose for anticoagulation. It slows the rate of thrombin production and inhibits its action. Intravascular coagulation is initiated by the slow release of tissue thromboplastin in some situations, or by the infusion of procoagulant as incompatible blood or prolonged extracorporeal bypass. The excess thrombin present converts the circulating fibrinogen to fibrin. Although hypofibrinogenemia is present, the administration of fibrinogen should not be started until the

"hypercoagulable state" has been corrected. After the intravascular coagulation has been adequately treated with heparin, hyperfibrinolysis may persist and then such antifibrinolysin therapy as Amicar or fibrinogen is indicated [68].

7 *Calcium gluconate* or *calcium chloride.* These drugs are sometimes given if there is evidence of hypocalcemia since calcium is necessary for the activation of prothrombin into thrombin (thrombin in turn transforms fibrinogen into fibrin). Most surgeons feel the patient can mobilize adequate calcium from his bones.

8 *Corticosteroids.* These are sometimes given in hypovolemic shock to improve tissue perfusion. The basis for their use comes from a theory that hypovolemic shock which persists will become less responsive to volume replacement because the reticuloendothelial system's ability to detoxify endotoxins in the intestinal tract is impaired. Absorption of these endotoxins results in endotoxic shock superimposed on hypovolemic shock [69]. Most of the rationale for the use of corticosteroids is based on experimentally bled animals treated with corticoids, but its use is encouraged if hypotension persists after the fluid volume has been replaced and any acidosis corrected [70].

Vasogenic (Septic) Shock

Vasogenic shock results in dilatation of the blood vessels and the loss of blood and plasma into the surrounding tissues. It is caused by such toxic substances as *histamine* and *endotoxins.* Histamine is produced as an allergic reaction to the administration of a drug or agent to which the patient had developed a hypersensitivity. Severe reactions are sometimes termed anaphylaxis. Endotoxins are produced by bacteria, especially gram-negative bacteria. Septicemia caused by gram-negative bacteria that is accompanied by shock is sometimes called gram-negative shock. It is not a frequent occurrence after open-heart surgery, but may result if a low-grade urinary infection flares up following trauma caused by passing a Foley catheter. A chronic infection in the lungs can also be activated by intubation, or the infection may be hospital-acquired when a portal of entry such as a urinary catheter, cutdown, or tracheostomy exists.

The symptoms that differ from the other types of shock also vary from patient to patient. In some cases, the onset and progression of symptoms is rapid, but in other cases the second stage may not appear for several hours or even several days [71]. The usual early symptoms are:

- Chills with fever to 101 to 104°F
- Skin warm and dry
- Normotension or hypotension
- Bradycardia
- Vomiting and diarrhea, which may include bloody stools

Later symptoms may include:

- Hypotension
- Skin moist and pale, with peripheral mottling and cyanosis
- Pulse weak and thready
- Peripheral veins collapsed
- Respirations rapid and shallow
- Decreased urinary output
- Hypothermia
- Convulsions and coma

Therapy

Therapy should be initiated promptly since endotoxic shock destroys as much microcirculation in minutes as usually occurs with hemorrhagic shock in hours [72]. Therapy includes:

- Culture and gram stain of the blood and all available sites of possible infection such as drainage from wound, urine, and cutdown catheter.
- Administration of large doses of broad-spectrum antibiotics. Kanamycin and penicillin are often given. As results of bacteriologic studies are available, antiobiotics may be changed to those that the infecting organism is sensitive to.
- Prompt administration of massive doses of corticosteroids. Most physicians prefer the glucocorticoid methylprednisolone (Solu-Medrol). Dosage of 125 mg to 1 gm may be repeated as often as every 2 hr. Some physicians feel a bolus does of 2 to 3 gm repeated in 12 to 24 hr is more beneficial. The corticoid is usually given in a single bolus dose and never continued more than 72 hr. Gastrointestinal bleeding, peptic ulceration, and uncontrollable

diabetes are the only known complications from massive administration of corticoids for a short period of time. The rationale
for the use of corticoid therapy is that in septic shock even though
the bacteria may be killed by antibiotics, the endotoxins will still
result in the pooling of blood in the extremities unless their
effect is counteracted. The hemodynamic effects of corticoid
therapy are:

1 Decreased peripheral resistance (Steroids deplete the store of
  norepinephrine in the postganglionic fibers and prevent spasm.)
2 Increased tissue perfusion
3 Increased venous return
4 Positive inotropic effect on the heart muscle
5 Since cortisone speeds up the conversion of glycogen to
  glucose in the liver, large doses result in a high blood sugar
  that needs to be carefully monitored.

- Cooling measures are indicated if temperature is elevated above
  101°F since elevation of temperature increases the metabolic
  requirements.
- Stabilization of the cardiovascular system by restoration of
  adequate circulating blood volume, and measures to correct
  accompanying heart failure and metabolic acidosis should be
  initiated when indicated.

HEART FAILURE

8

Heart failure is the term used to describe the inability of the heart adequately to pump out all the blood that returns to it. This results in blood backing up in the chambers of the heart, in the pulmonary system, and in the veins that return blood to the heart. The hydrostatic pressure created by the backing up of blood in the blood vessels forces fluid out of the vessels into the extracellular spaces in the lungs, legs, abdomen, and other areas. Heart failure also causes a diminished renal blood flow because of the decrease in cardiac output, which causes sodium to be retained by the kidney. The retention of sodium also necessitates the retention of water, which results in a build-up of excess sodium and water in the extracellular compartment.

Heart failure is usually ascribed as failure of either the right or the left ventricle of the heart, although both are often present to some degree.

RIGHT-SIDED HEART FAILURE

The fluid backs up into the veins of the systemic circulation causing edema of the extremities, ascites, hepatomegaly, distended neck veins, and similar conditions. If the heart failure is secondary to disorders of the lungs and/or pulmonary arteries, it is termed *cor pulmonale*. The obstruction or impairment to breathing raises the pressure in the pulmonary arteries, which requires the right ventricle to work harder to overcome the increase in pulmonary artery pressure. The increased work causes the right ventricle to become enlarged and right heart failure results, preventing the right ventricle from ejecting all its blood. As the ventricle fails, central venous engorgement occurs and the tissue capillary pressure rises above the blood colloid osmotic pressure, causing interstitial edema. Although cor pulmonale may be caused by chronic obstructive disease of the lung or by pulmonary valvular insufficiency and stenosis, the sudden onset of cor pulmonale in the postoperative heart patient is usually caused by occlusion of a major pulmonary vessel by a massive pulmonary embolus.

LEFT-SIDED HEART FAILURE

The fluid accumulates in the pulmonary veins and progresses to the alveolar spaces. *Acute pulmonary edema* caused by left-sided heart failure is a medical emergency since if it is not immediately treated, the patient may drown in his own secretions. It may result from dislodgment of a heart valve prosthesis, rapid overreplacement of blood, plasma, or blood volume expanders, or failure of the ventricle. Extreme anxiety may be a contributing factor.

Acute pulmonary edema can usually be distinguished from a pulmonary embolus by the following diagnostic criteria:

Symptom	Acute Pulmonary Edema	Pulmonary Embolus
Feeling of apprehension and suffocation	Yes	Moderate
Tachycardia	Yes	Yes
Ventricular gallop rhythm	Yes	No
Tachypnea	Yes	Yes
Dyspnea	Yes	Yes
Cyanosis	Peripheral usually	15% of the time
Cough	Yes	50% of the time
Frothy hemoptysis	Yes, in advanced stage	25% of the time
Severe pleuritic pain	No	35 to 50% of the time
Cold, sweaty skin	Yes	Yes
LDH (lactic dehydrogenase)	Normal (25–100 units)	Elevated 90% of the time
Lung infiltrate	Yes	No

Symptom	Acute Pulmonary Edema	Pulmonary Embolus
Blood pressure	Initially elevated, then hypotensive	Hypotension
Positive jugular reflux (distension of neck veins when the liver is depressed)	No	Yes
Wheezing and rhonchi, rales	Yes, in advanced cases	Yes, usually
Temperature above 99°F	No	Elevated 55% of the time

Treatment

The main goal of treatment and the methods used to accomplish this goal for either heart failure with pulmonary edema or pulmonary embolus is to improve pulmonary ventilation and oxygen saturation. This is best accomplished by:

- The use of a respirator. One hundred percent oxygen may be needed. Fourteen to fifteen liters of oxygen a minute need to be given if a respirator is not available.

- Ethyl alcohol, 50 to 95 percent, is frequently used in the nebulizer for its antifoaming effect to reduce the respiratory obstruction resulting from the mechanical interference of edema fluid.

- The use of bronchodilators such as aminophylline or papaverine parenterally to reduce bronchospasm. Epinephrine and isoproterenol (Isuprel) may be given by nebulizer.

- The administration of morphine intravenously to reduce pulmonary congestion, relieve dyspnea, and reduce anxiety.

- Elevation of the head of the bed 60 to 90 degrees to allow for full pulmonary expansion and to decrease the intrapulmonary blood volume.

- To conserve the oxygen needs by controlling the patient's activities such as not serving him large meals; preventing constipation and discouraging straining at stools; spacing nursing activities throughout the day to allow the patient periods of uninterrupted rest; and reducing excessive anxiety.

Therapy for pulmonary embolus also includes:

- The use of *anticoagulants* to limit propagation of clots. Heparin is usually given with an initial dose of 5000 units intravenously. Heparin is considered to have a thrombolytic action that helps dissolve old clots although most physicians feel it does not affect clots more than 24 hr old. Postoperative patients who still have chest tubes need to be carefully evaluated before heparin is used. The use of fibrolytic enzymes (e.g., fibrinolysin) is still experimental and results are inconclusive.

- The use of elastic stockings on the extremities to prevent further thrombus or embolus formation.

- Pulmonary artery embolectomy may be attempted, although the use of the heart-lung bypass machine is hazardous (Fig. 8–1). New techniques are being developed to remove the embolus without the use of the bypass procedure, but they are still in the experimental stage.

- Ligation of the inferior vena cava may be done to prevent further pulmonary emboli.

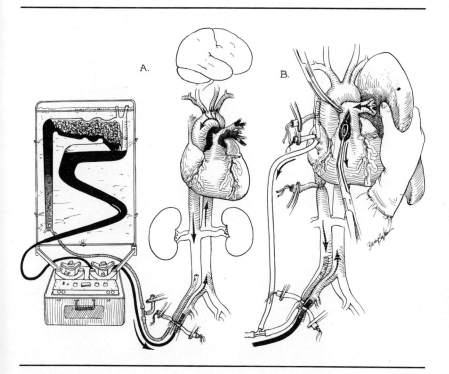

FIGURE 8–1 Technique of pulmonary embolectomy using cardiopulmonary bypass. (A) depicts cannulation of femoral artery and vein for initial partial bypass; (B) depicts total cardiopulmonary bypass with embolus removal.

Treatment for pulmonary edema also includes:

- *Diuretics* to increase sodium and water excretion. The most effective drugs are furosemide (Lasix) and ethracrynic acid (Edecrin). They are usually given intravenously.
- *Restriction of sodium and fluid.*[1]
- *Rotating tourniquets*, sometimes termed a bloodless phlebotomy. Tourniquets are applied so arterial blood may enter the extremity, but venous flow from it is slowed. Since blood is pooled in the extremities, less blood is returned to the heart. An electrical tourniquet machine increases the effectiveness of the process. The tourniquet should be placed as high on the extremity as possible. When manual tourniquets are used, one tourniquet should be rotated in a clockwise pattern to the free limb at least every 15 min. The peripheral pulse in the extremity needs to be checked frequently to ensure that arterial circulation is not compromised. When tourniquets are discontinued, only one tourniquet should be removed every 15 min so that pooled blood is released in small amounts.
- *Phlebotomy* of 250 to 500 cc of blood to decrease the blood volume rapidly may be done on patients with intractable pulmonary edema.
- *Digitalis* is given to improve the pumping action of the heart. If the patient has not been receiving digitalis, a full digitalizing dose of a rapid acting form of digitalis such as ouabain or deslanoside (Cedilanid D) may be used. Since digitalis preparations cause a fall in left ventricular end diastolic pressure, they lessen the degree of pulmonary congestion.

[1]Electrolyte determinations of plasma may misrepresent conditions in other spaces. The plasma of an edematous cardiac patient may show a reduced serum sodium concentration despite an enormous excess of total body sodium. This is because in severe heart failure, on a low-sodium diet, water may be retained in excess of sodium. This dilutes the concentration of all electrolytes in body fluids.

EMBOLIZATION

9

CAUSES OF EMBOLI

An embolus is an abnormal material circulating in the blood stream which becomes lodged in some vessel that is too small to permit its passage. Common embolic sites are the lungs, brain, coronary arteries, mesentery, limbs, kidney, and spleen. An embolus may be caused by a blood clot or thrombus, air, fat globules, a clump of bacteria, a piece of tissue, or a calcium plaque.

Blood clot emboli may result from dislodgement of a mural thrombus during surgery, dislodgement of a clot on a valve, venous stasis, injury to the intima of the blood vessels, or from alterations in coagulability following surgery. Symptoms of occlusion of a vessel by a clot are related to the area of occlusion and to the adequacy of the collateral circulation. Emboli to the brain may give symptoms similar to those of cerebrovascular accident (CVA). Symptoms may include weakness on one side or of upper extremities, changes in pupil reaction and size, and a bilateral Hoffmann's reaction. Pulmonary embolism has been discussed under right-sided heart failure, or cor pulmonale.

Arterial blood clots may block the carotid, femoral, renal, mesenteric, and other arteries. When they lodge in a major artery, they may be fatal or result in permanent damage.

A *mesenteric embolus* is fatal unless diagnosis and surgical intervention to resect all necrotic bowel and restore bowel blood supply are initiated promptly. The symptoms are severe, sudden midabdominal and/or midback pain; moderate abdominal distension; vomiting and loose blood-tinged stools; diaphoresis; and progressive development of shock. The diagnostic aids are leukocytosis to 20,000 cells per cu ml; x-ray demonstration of scattered small amounts of gas; arteriography by retrograde catheter which shows obstruction; and sigmoidoscopy, which shows ischemia and/or necrosis of the intestinal mucosa.

Treatment is surgical embolectomy and resection of all necrotic bowel with anastomosis or temporary exteriorization of bowel ends. With early restoration of blood flow, extensive bowel resection may be avoided [73].

Emboli to an artery of the extremities may result in loss of the extremity if adequate treatment is not quickly given. Signs and symptoms are severe sudden pain at site of emboli; cessation of pulses in extremity; nausea and vomiting; whiteness, coldness, blotching, tingling, and numbness of extremity; and progressive development of shock and cyanosis of extremity, with development of gangrene if collateral circulation is inadequate.

Treatment is an embolectomy done within a few hours while the extremities are still viable. Emboli at any point from the aorta to the ankle can be removed through the femoral artery. The best indicators of viability are preservation of the sensation of light touch, and presence of capillary blanching with the application of pressure. If gangrene is present or viability is seriously impaired, an amputation will have to be done.

The aim of other measures in the interim before surgery is to improve the general condition and prevent further damage. If not contraindicated by the patient's general condition, other measures may include:

- Anticoagulants to prevent further propagation of the clot. Heparin may have a slight thrombolytic action as well as preventing further clots.

- Vasodilating drugs to improve the collateral circulation.

- Careful wrapping of ischemic extremity with a sterile cotton blanket and the use of a foot cradle to protect the extremity from injury.

- Use of low molecular weight dextran (LMWD) (a rheologic agent with a molecular weight of 40,000) in place of anticoagulants, which seems to have the following beneficial effects: relieves ischemic pain, reverses anesthesia, maintains distal artery patency, prevents red cell aggregation, and improves microcirculation [74]. LMWD must be given cautiously to avoid circulatory overload as it is a volume expander. It is eliminated by the kidneys in 6 to 8 hr so dosages must be repeated to maintain effect. Usual dosage is 500 ml of 10 percent solution every 6 hr.

• Use of fibrolytic agents to dissolve clots has sometimes proved effective, but the management of patients receiving the drugs has been difficult, and it is hard to maintain blood concentrations high enough to alter the rate of clot lysis. The most commonly used agents are Actase and Thrombolysin. They should be started within 24 hr for greatest effectiveness, and thrombi older than 72 hr are resistant to lysis. Administration may produce fever and there is a high incidence of allergic reactions. Urokinase is a newer fibrolytic agent being tested that looks promising, but at the present time is very expensive [75].

Air emboli can occur after open-heart surgery because the cardiac chambers are open and air may be trapped in the left or right side of the heart. Air in the left side of the heart is most serious as it not only results in myocardial ischemia, which may prevent the heart from resuming normal contractions after defibrillation, but it may also go to the brain and result in brain damage. To prevent air emboli, the atrium and ventricle are vented and air forced out of the heart before discontinuance of bypass. Sometimes a needle in the aorta is used to aspirate any residual air. The damage caused by an air embolus is usually more transient than that caused by a blood clot. Symptomatic treatment may include the use of anticonvulsants when indicated; maintenance of normothermia to reduce the metabolic rate and oxygen requirements; the administration of oxygen by a respirator to prevent unnecessary tissue hypoxia; and prevention of cerebral edema.

Fat emboli may result from particles of bone marrow broken off when the sternum is split; the particles are forced into the vascular system by the high interstitial pressure in the bone, and fat globules that result from the alteration of normal lipid stability that accompanies the trauma to the red blood cells during long cardiopulmonary bypass procedure. Blood clots are retained by the filter, but fat globules pass through the filter. Fat emboli may also result from cardiac compression with trauma to the sternum.

The lung is the organ mainly affected by fat emboli, but fat globules can pass through the pulmonary vessels and cause peripheral embolization, especially in the brain. The clinical signs are: (a) dyspnea and cyanosis, with a rapid respiratory rate of 30 to 46; (b) moist pulmonary rales with persistent cough; (c) tachycardia of 140; (d) temperature rise as high as 103°F; (e) restlessness, disorientation, lethargy, and possibly delirium; (f) sometimes presence of decerebrate rigidity; (g) petechial rash, which may appear on the second or third day over upper trunk, axillae, and conjunctivae; (h) laboratory findings, which are time-consuming and occasionally misleading, of fat globules in the urine and elevated serum lipase; (i) chest x-ray findings, which may demonstrate a "snow-storm" appearance with the loss of vascular markings and diffuse parenchymal infiltrate similar to pulmonary edema although vascular congestion and pleural effusion are absent.

The treatment may include

Prevention of tissue hypoxia by use of oxygen by a respirator

The use of heparin in small amounts (1000 to 5000 units) every 6 to 8 hr—results are equivocal

The use of corticosteroids, of debatable beneficial effect

The use of low molecular weight dextran when it is not contraindicated

Symptomatic treatment of any accompanying shock [76]

NURSING ASSESSMENT

Nursing assessment includes observation of any signs of emboli. Routine checks should be made hourly for the first 24 hr postoperatively of:

Level of consciousness and ability to respond to verbal commands

Pupil reaction and size

Recognition of painful stimuli

Ability to move all extremities

Strength of handgrip

Presence of peripheral pulses

Color and warmth of extremities

Signs of respiratory insufficiency such as dyspnea, cough, and tachypnea if patient is not on the respirator

Ability to speak if not intubated

NURSING PREVENTION OF AN EMBOLUS

- Use of antiembolic stockings or leg wraps to increase the flow of blood in the deep veins, thus reducing the danger of venous stasis. If Ace wraps are used instead of stockings, they should be applied so there is no zone of tight constriction and the pressure is high at the foot and gradually decreases to the knee. The stockings or wraps should be removed twice a day for 10 or 15 min.

- Use of active and passive range of motion exercises to prevent loss of muscle tone and provide muscular pressure on the veins to assist the return flow of blood to the heart. Dorsiflexion of the ankles is especially important since it stretches the muscles in the calves of the legs.

- Keeping the knee gatch on the bed flat, avoiding the use of pillows under the knees, and discouraging any crossing of the legs since pressure on the popliteal space where vessels are superficial may predispose to thrombus formation.

- Early ambulation, but limitation of periods of sitting in a chair. If patient's condition prevents him from ambulation by the fourth postoperative day, it is sometimes advisable to transfer him to a CircOlectric bed so he can be placed in an upright position with weight-bearing on his feet several times a day.

NURSING CARE

1 Careful observation for any change in condition
2 Patience and empathetic understanding of anxiety and discouragement the patient may be experiencing with explanation geared to the patient's level of understanding
3 Care in moving patient to avoid dislodgement of emboli
4 Care and protection of any portion of the body with a reduced blood supply, e.g., lamb's wool between toes, boot, cradle, and sterile cotton blanket wrap of legs

REACTIONS TO STRESS

10

Patients with any kind of illness experience both physiological and psychological stress. Open-heart surgery has an especially strong emotional impact because of the symbolic importance of the heart as "the vital organ" and because the surgery requires the heart to be stopped temporarily and perhaps permanently. The way the patient reacts to the threatening ordeal of surgery largely depends on

His past life experiences, which have conditioned him to react in specific ways.

The degree or extent of the preoperative incapacity.

The emotional resources of the patient to maintain stability in the presence of stress, which is sometimes referred to as the "integrative capacity."

His level of acceptance of his heart condition with integration of it into his self-concept and the pattern of his life.

Existence of unresolved stress preoperatively, which could be caused by failure in interpersonal relations or failure to achieve goals.

Degree of flexibility in ideals of behavior. Patients with rigid and exacting ideals are more vulnerable to psychological complications when they are unable to maintain their ideal behavior.

Magnitude of new stress patient is subjected to.

The relationship of the patient to the physicians and nurses.

Stress activates the homeostatic process known as the sympatho-adrenal response, which includes increased stimulation of the sympathetic nervous system to produce norepinephrine and the increased secretion of adrenocorticosteriod hormones. Although this response is a protective mechanism to help the person escape the stress-producing situation or mobilize his defenses to resist it, the effects of the sympathoadrenal response may tax the cardiovascular system and adversely affect the postoperative course. Therefore it is important for the nurse to observe behavioral manifestations of increasing stress, and to explore forces operating in nursing situations that contribute to the development of stress.

PHYSIOLOGICAL MANIFESTATIONS

These may vary, depending on the general condition of the patient, but some usual physiological reactions are:

- Laboratory measurements, which include increase in serum cate-cholamines, increase in eosinophils, increased excretion of cortico-steroids and catecholamines in the urine, and retention of sodium in the body.
- Elevation of blood pressure.
- Increase in heart and respiratory rate.
- Increase in perspiration.
- Dryness of mouth.
- Inhibition of peristalsis.
- Changes in the mucous membrane (especially of the gas-trointestinal tract), which may include engorgement, ischemia, hemorrhage, edema, erosion, ulceration, and inflammation. The development of a stress ulcer that frequently hemorrhages is one of the most common manifestations of mucous membrane change [77].

PSYCHOLOGICAL MANIFESTATIONS

Signs may be anxiety, decrease in level of cognitive functioning, depression, confusion, and delirium. Each manifestation will be discussed, but since the treatment or prevention includes many common factors, the common apsects of the nursing approach will be considered at the end.

Anxiety

Anxiety is a complex unpleasant emotional reaction to stress and the threat to one's self-concept. Frieda Fromm termed anxiety "The most unpleasant, and at the same time, the most universal experience except loneliness." Feelings of powerlessness, isolation, and insecurity often underlie the experience of anxiety. The degree of anxiety a patient experiences depends on how he perceives and interprets the situation. His behavioral response to anxiety depends on the patterns he has already formed as a result of cultural and operant conditioning, on his level of maturity, and on the behavior of significant others in his environment.

Defense Mechanisms

If the situation is too threatening for the patient to face, he may use a defense mechanism to reduce conscious awareness of the anxiety-producing situation, thus making it easier for him to cope with the situation. Each individual develops his own means of meeting anxiety and relieving tension. It is important that the nurse does not just observe and respond to the behavior exhibited by the patient, but finds the cause for the behavior. If a certain defense mechanism is the best method a patient has for controlling anxiety, then it should be maintained and encouraged in the critical period.

Defense mechanisms that the individual may use to escape the reality and thus reduce anxiety according to Dennis [78] are aggression—moving against others in the situation; overdependency—moving toward others in the situation; or withdrawal—moving away from the situation.

Aggression

Aggression may be a patient's way of reacting to a stressful situation. It can be understood since anger and resentment toward the persons responsible for the stressful situation is a normal reaction. Male patients especially are prone to hide their anxiety by aggressive action, since it is more acceptable to them to be hostile than admit to fear and anxiety. A patient who is accustomed to reacting to stress with aggression may have conflicts during the critical stage of his illness when he is so dependent on others that he is fearful of retaliation or rejection if he gives expression to his feeling that he is not understood, appreciated, or cared for adequately. Since repression of hostility generates more anxiety, the nurse must help the patient understand and handle his hostility. One method is to put what she knows must be his thoughts into words, such as "I know you must get terribly tired of us continually asking you to cough, but it is important for you to keep your lungs clear." Since our normal way of reacting to hostility or aggression is defensive in an attempt to satisfy our own feelings, it sometimes takes a great deal of practice for the nurse to learn to focus on the patient's feelings rather than her own and to encourage the patient to express his hostile feelings.

Overdependency

Overdependency is a less frequently noted defense mechanism, possibly because the open-heart surgery patient is so dependent on others during his critical period. Most patients are able to accept their position of physical helplessness as a justifiable limitation resulting from their surgery rather than as a sign of personal weakness or inadequacy. After the critical period is past, they can relinquish the dependency that was forced upon them and return to their previous patterns of behavior. A few individuals who have been rigidly self-sufficient and independent before surgery may shift to the other extreme and exhibit exaggerated dependence and helplessness following surgery. The patient may always have had underlying dependent needs and his insistence on independence was a reaction to keep him from giving in to dependency and losing his self-esteem. Although the patient has to accept dependence during the critical period, he needs to be encouraged to assist in the decisions and his care as much as possible, and his attention needs to be directed to what he will be able to do in the future to prevent him from slipping into a pattern of dependent chronic psychological invalidism.

Withdrawal

Withdrawal is the defense mechanism most often used during the first 48 hours after open-heart surgery. It is difficult to assess how much is psychological and how much is physiological. Men seem to be especially prone to withdraw, possibly because the image of themselves with no control over the situation and dependent on others for all their needs is too distressing for them to handle, especially when it is coupled with the fear that they may not live. Withdrawal may actually be beneficial in the early postoperative period because it reduces the response to stimuli that might result in a sensory overload that would tax the cardiovascular system and the integrative capacity of the patient. However, the nurse should try to keep the lines of communication open so the patient maintains some contact with reality and has an opportunity to express himself if he desires. Apathy is to be avoided since it reduces the motivation to recover.

Decrease in Level of Cognitive Functioning

The decrease is evident by a lowered ability accurately to perceive and interpret stimuli. The patient with severe cognitive limitations may exhibit centering (taking into account and focusing on only one aspect of the situation) or egocentric representations (inability to see any conclusion other than his own, or to give any justification to support his viewpoint). Although primarily psychological, the cognitive level may also be affected by physiological states such as fatigue and response to the administration of drugs that decrease the patient's perception of his environment and his level of mental functioning.

Schlesinger [79] describes three major disorders in reception of stimuli:

1 *Distractibility.* The inability to direct the train of thought or attention on relevant stimuli, with the result that thought is aimlessly influenced by chance stimuli.

2 *Hypovigilance.* A reduction in the number of stimuli received with a delay in response to stimuli. An extreme example is somnolence in which virtually no stimuli are received.

3 *Hypervigilance.* Undue susceptibility to stimuli, which may be exhibited by either *(a)* tenacity of attention, in which the attention is so focused on the first stimulus that subsequent stimuli are either ignored or responded to slowly, or *(b)* shifting vigilance, in which the attention shifts rapidly from one stimulus to another. It may be accompanied by restless movements and extreme irritability.

Psychological factors that contribute to a decrease in the level of cognitive functioning are

1   The feeling of powerlessness that leads the patient to believe that he has no control over his situation and that his behavior will have no influence on the outcome he seeks.

2   Lack of knowledge and understanding of his postoperative plan of care, the medical terminology that he hears, and the equipment.

3   Inability to maintain an optimal level of varying forms of sensory input which, according to Solomon [80], results in perceptual deprivation, which is an absence of any pattern to which meaning can be ascribed; perceptual monotony; and sensory overload.

Depression

Depression is an emotional condition characterized by discouragement, sense of futility, feelings of inadequacy, and a decrease in functional activity. When the patient has successfully come through his surgery and is progressing normally, the usual response is relief and sometimes a mild euphoria at having "made it." (It is important to remember, however, that euphoria is sometimes an attempt to deny depression.) If complications develop, the patient is faced with the fearful possibility that he may die. When the self-image he had of himself successfully recovering from surgery is threatened, he tends to assume that because his concept of himself is altered, others will lose their esteem and affection for him also. Depression is a method of expressing these negative feelings. Sometimes the patient uses withdrawal, depersonalization, or denial to avoid accepting the situation. The value of these defense mechanisms is limited, because they usually cannot be successfully maintained and the patient eventually has to face the reality of the situation. The nurse needs to demonstrate to the patient that she respects him and then help him to explore, identify, and accept his feelings of depression as legitimate feelings, before she can find him receptive to accepting realistically the positive aspects of his condition.

Confusion and Delirium

These symptoms may be an extension of the other manifestations of stress that have not been adequately controlled. In a study of 119 adult cardiac surgery patients, 38 percent of the patients experienced at least some manifestations of a psychosis-like syndrome that began after a lucid interval of 3 to 5 days and sometimes lasted 14 days [81]. Other studies have found that as high as 57 percent of the open-heart surgery patients developed a psychosis that is sometimes termed post-cardiotomy delirium [82]. Disordered thinking, perceptual distortions, visual illusions or hallucinations, and disorientation to time, place, and person were the most frequent manifestations.

CAUSATIVE FACTORS OF PSYCHOSIS

The factors responsible for the psychosis are related to the patient himself, to various aspects of his treatment, and to his environment. *Factors related to the patient*, which seem to increase the incidence, are

1 Preoperative problems, especially those that pertain to unsettled interpersonal relationships
2 Preoperative existence of an organic brain syndrome or severe cardiac decompensation
3 Use of large doses of barbiturates or heavy ingestion of alcohol over a fairly long period of time before surgery, which can result in delirium from withdrawal

Although preoperative psychiatric disorder is related to increased mortality rate, it was found to be unrelated to incidence of psychosis [82].

Factors related to the treatment, which Dr. Blachly [82] found significantly increased the incidence of psychosis, are

1 Longer anesthesia than 6 hr.
2 Pump bypass run 2 hr or longer. When pump run was 4 hr, 100 percent of the patients developed delirium, although some other studies failed to confirm this correlation.
3 No blood at all or more than 15 units of blood given.
4 Hypothermia more than 6 degrees below 37°C.
5 Dehydration with low serum sodium and magnesium [83].

The mechanisms by which cardiopulmonary bypass and hypothermia damage the central nervous system suggested by Dr. Blachly [82] are

1 Alteration of serum proteins by the bypass machine

2 EEG abnormalities resulting from inadequate cerebral perfusion

3 Lodging of microemboli in cerebral capillaries

4 Releasing of serotonin and related substances from the platelets as the steroid level falls

Factors related to the environment, which seem to increase the incidence of psychosis, are

1 Abnormal sensory input, with lack of variety or meaningfulness of the stimuli and absence of familiar sights and sounds (Fig. 10–1).

2 Sleep deprivation, with periods of delirium being preceded by one or two sleepless nights.

3 Auditory EKG monitoring. In some patients EEG changes have been recorded after only 6 to 30 min of hearing one click every second [84].

4 Monotonous rhythmic noise of the respirator.

5 Immobilization from apparatus or restraints, which prevents adequate kinesthetic stimulation.

6 Presence of aura of disaster.

7 Loss of orientation to date and time.

8 Impersonal attitude of staff, and excessive limitations on visits from family.

NURSING INTERVENTION

Nursing intervention to prevent or reduce psychological reactions to stress includes the development and maintenance of a *therapeutic relationship* that will undergird and help sustain the patient during the stressful surgical period and will promote his personal growth toward effective handling of his own problems. In a therapeutic relationship the nurse acts as an ego surrogate for the patient while his strength is depleted by illness. Some factors that promote a therapeutic relationship are:

• Accurate and continuing assessment of the patient's feelings that result from the stress. Jourard uses the term *disclosure* to describe the act of communicating these feelings [85]. Communication can be both verbal and nonverbal. Nonverbal communication may

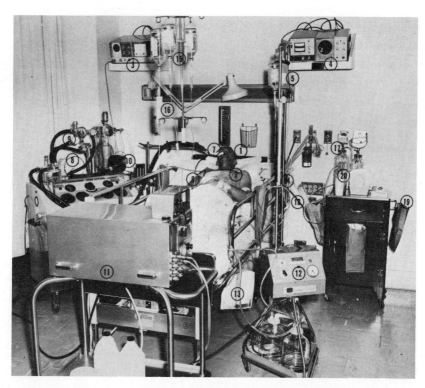

FIGURE 10–1 The environment of the intensive care unit with its many machines can be a source of stress. Depicted are: (1) patient 24 hr after aortic valve replacement; (2) EKG monitoring leads on chest; (3) EKG oscilloscope and heart rate meter; (4) central arterial pressure wave form and read out meters; (5) arterial pressure infusor bag with transfer pack containing heparinized solution for maintaining patency of the arterial line; (6) sphygmomanometer with blood pressure cuff for comparison measurement; (7) endotracheal tube with tubing from Engstrom respirator connected; (8) spirometer on Engstrom respirator for measuring expired minute volume; (9) airway pressure gauge, which shows pressure that is required to deliver volume of air and oxygen; (10) Ambu bag for manual sighing or for use in power failure; (11) hypothermia machine with reserve supply of alcohol solution; (12) Emerson suction for chest tube drainage; (13) Cystoflow bag for urinary drainage; (14) CVP manometer; (15) IV fluid administration system; (16) buretrol for addition of antibiotics to IV line; (17) suction for endotracheal suctioning; (18) sterile catheters for endotracheal suctioning; (19) bag for soiled suction catheters; and (20) sterile saline and cups for suctioning use.

reveal a patient's hidden thoughts and feelings and includes the use of gestures, body movements, and changes in inflections and tone of voice. Nonverbal communication often gives an indication of an area that needs to be explored with the patient. Since the patient suffers a feeling of isolation that further increases his stress when his feelings cannot be communicated to others, the nurse needs to be skillful in promoting communication [85]. Some techniques to facilitate verbal communication are:

(1) Make a statement about the patient's behavior as you see it and ask the patient to verify that it is true. "It seems to me that you are fighting going to sleep. Is this true?"

(2) Encourage the patient to continue talking by repeating what the patient said. "You say you are afraid to fall asleep."

(3) Ask another question to clarify what has been said. "Do you feel that you are more apt to have a serious complication develop when you're asleep than when you are awake?"

(4) Use of open-end statements or questions for the patient to complete. "And by staying awake you feel you will be able to . . .?"

(5) Interject another problem that may help the patient gain insight to the present problem. "How do you feel that it will help if you remain awake?"

(6) Reflect the feeling you think the patient has. "It must be a terrible feeling to know you need to sleep but not to be able to let go."

- Eye contact, honest answers rather than evasions, and language that the patient understands promote communication. The patient should be given time to respond. If the patient does not answer when the nurse attempts to explore his feelings, it is helpful for the nurse to acknowledge that there are some feelings that are too difficult to put into words, but she thinks she understands how he feels and that she will sit quietly beside him for a while. Placing her hand on top of the patient's or lightly stroking his forehead communicates her concern.

- Acceptance of the patient as he is without being judgmental or making an evaluation from one's own viewpoint. Acceptance of the patient reduces the need for the patient to be defensive about his behavior and thus it makes it easier for him to accept his own feelings and work toward any necessary changes.

- Maintenance of an environment in which each patient retains a sense of personal worth and dignity. This includes (1) avoidance of any unnecessary exposure or embarrassment; (2) introduction to new personnel; and (3) use of the patient's name. Asking the patient preoperatively how he pronounces his name, and what name he would like the nurses to call him helps to have the first-name basis used for only those patients who have stated it as their preference.

- Demonstration of genuine concern and esteem for the patient. Any effort to get to know the feelings of the patient without caring about him can be cruel and destructive. The humanistic caring for the patient transforms the cold environment dominated by machines into an environment centered on concern for the patient.

- Reenforcement of the patient's belief in something or someone. Some patients find hope and assurance from their religious beliefs.

- Recognition of the importance of the patient's family. Whether the family's presence is therapeutic for the patient or contraindicated must be carefully evaluated. Sometimes the family may need help in handling their own feelings and time to regain their composure. If the nurse can channel the family's fear and anxiety into identification and realistic solutions of their concerns and problems, the patient will benefit.

- Response of the nurse matched to the emotional intensity of the patient. The patient's concerns need to be accepted as legitimate concerns rather than to be lightly dismissed or responded to by a humorous remark.

- It has been the experience of the author that the use of Turner's concept of the interactive, nonreflexive role-taking is extremely useful in establishing a therapeutic relationship. "Role" is defined as a "collection of patterns of behavior that are thought to constitute a meaningful unit and deemed appropriate." Interactive role-taking is the process of engaging in the imaginative construction of the role of another while examining the probable interaction between the self-role and the other-role in terms of promotion of a purpose, and shaping one's own role behavior according to what one judges to be the probable effect of interaction between one's own role and the inferred role of the other. "Nonreflexive" directs attention to attitudes in the role of the other whose recognition makes it possible to act according to the purpose, rather than manipulation of the self-image for the means of achieving the purpose [86]. When this concept is applied to the patient situation, it enables the nurse to understand, accept, and support the patient's attitudes and psychological adaptive mechanisms toward his illness. The interaction will modify the nurse's conception and performance of her own role, so that the nursing intervention she designs and implements will reflect the desires and needs of the patient and help him accept his state of illness. This concept embodies empathy but it goes further in that it helps the nurse to be sensitive to the patient's needs and to modify her own behavior so that the patient knows she is sensitive and concerned about his feelings.

Other measures to reduce psychological reactions to stress are:

- *Increasing the knowledge and understanding* of the patient. Preoperative teaching is important, but explanations frequently need to be repeated postoperatively. All explanations should be geared to the patient's level of understanding. Since there is a danger of increasing anxiety when the patient is given inappropriate information, or since information can be misinterpreted, the nurse can increase her effectiveness by first asking the patient what he has been told.

- *Giving the patient more control* in the situation by allowing him to participate in the decision-making process whenever possible. During the first few days, it is difficult to let the patient feel he has any control. However, asking him if he feels he needs medication for pain, which side he wants to be turned on, if he would like to have the light dimmed, or if he wants the head of his bed raised or lowered does reduce the feeling of powerlessness. Nite found that bringing the patient into the treatment plan helped him gain an insight into what his future activities would include and he then showed less concern about the future and fewer expressions of depression [87].

- *Fostering trust* in the patient that he is in the hands of competent persons who will be able to care for all his needs. Faith in the healing ability of the staff serves as a psychological bulwark during the early period of acute stress [88]. The patient gains confidence in the nursing staff when the various members are consistent in their method of giving treatments, measuring parameters, and operating equipment. Any discussions of pros and cons of treatment or differences of opinion should be conducted away from the patient's bedside. When the nurse is able to hide her own anxiety, talking unhurriedly with the patient while avoiding any bustling activity, both the patient and the family will feel more secure. Being always readily available when needed assures the patient that he will not be left unattended.

- *Alleviating pain,* which is discussed under a separate section, is important in the reduction of stress.

- *Preventing undue fatigue* by arranging for the patient to have some uninterrupted periods of sleep. Use of comfort measures such as a soothing light rub of the lower back, wiping the face with a cool cloth, and a refreshing mouthwash.

- *Controlling abnormal sensory states* by (a) Reorienting patient to time, place, and person. A clock and a calendar within patient's line of vision are helpful. (b) Providing patient with his glasses, hearing aid, or wristwatch. (c) Assigning the same personnel to care for the patient for several successive days, if possible. (d) Using such familiar objects at bedside as family pictures, small radio, his own toilet articles. (e) Providing for tactile and kinesthetic stimulation through back rub, position changes, and exercises of legs and arms to lessen the stress of enforced immobility. The use of a bean bag larger than a pillow is being explored by the author as a means of giving the patient an outlet for his aggressive feelings and physical exercise. Since physical activity reduces the sympathoadrenal response to stress, it serves to reduce the effects of stress as well as the cause of stress. (f) Using disk leads for EKG monitoring and keeping the right hand free so the patient can write when he is intubated, which helps to keep immobilization at a minimum. (g) Avoiding such meaningless stimuli that can be misinterpreted or create stress as the audible "beep" or "click" of the EKG machine, shadows from poor lighting of equipment areas, and so on. (h) Using a unit designed in such a way that there are outside windows to help with orientation and maintenance of a feeling of reality. (i) Providing an interesting visual background.

- *Instituting such measures to modify confusion and delirium* as (a) giving support and protection to a patient during confused behavior; (b) use of restraints to keep patient from harming himself; (c) recognition that hallucinations are inappropriate, accompanied by assurances that they are quite common and normal; and (d) use of phenothiazines such as Thorazine and Mellaril for moderate or severe confusion or delirium.

- *Providing motivation for recovery.* The nurse is sometimes the person who is present when the patient becomes disheartened and is ready to give up. Realistic hopeful reassurance will sometimes give him the lift he needs to continue to fight. Sometimes enumerating the positive aspects of his progress will rekindle the motivation to live. A patient who had been on the respirator for four days with a postperfusion syndrome following the placement of an aortic valve prosthesis exhibited marked apathy. When he was shown his chest x-ray of the aortic valve and was reassured that although he felt he wasn't getting enough oxygen, his valve was working perfectly and his lungs would gradually improve, his behavior markedly improved and he did recover.

When anxiety persists beyond the critical period, the nurse can help the patient identify his anxiety, gain insight into the cause for the anxiety, and cope with his feelings. The use of a guided problem-solving approach in which the nurse helps the patient explore his feelings and reasons for his behavior but allows him to formulate his own plan for coping with the situation is one of the most effective ways of helping him. The nurse's attitude that the patient will be able to recognize the cause of his anxiety and handle it increases his confidence in his own ability.

In order for the nurse to be effective in meeting the emotional needs of the patient, she must understand and be able to control her own emotional reactions, so that she does not communicate her anxiety, or other emotions, to the patient. One of the most difficult aspects for the intensive care nurse, who sometimes must make a decision that may mean life or death for the patient, is to learn to live realistically with the fear that she may make an error. Unless she has accepted the fact of human fallibility, her fear will hinder her effectiveness in a crisis situation.

In order for the nurse to make the emotional commitment necessary to provide the care the patient needs, her own psychological and social needs must be met. Brown [89] has identified the following needs of the nursing personnel: social approval, sense of accomplishment, sense of importance of the job, security, and, support in anxiety-inducing situations.

When the organizational structure of the intensive care unit recognizes the potential within each nurse and encourages growth, provides guidance, fosters involvement in decision-making, creates opportunities, removes obstacles, and acknowledges the contribution of each individual, the environment is conducive to the development of therapeutic relationships.

ELECTROLYTE AND ACID-BASE PROBLEMS

11

Although abnormal electrolyte concentrations can cause many problems, the two most common problems are hyponatremic syndrome and hypokalemic metabolic alkalosis.

POSTCOMMISSUROTOMY HYPONATREMIC SYNDROME

This is the term given to a sodium deficit that develops following heart operations, especially those for mitral stenosis. The probable cause is the cessation of the preoperative atrial distension, resulting in hypersecretion of ADH with retention of water and the dilution of the body fluids, and producing a "dilutional hyponatremia." This condition is sometimes referred to as water intoxication. If water overloading develops rapidly or is severe, the patient may develop symptoms such as disturbed thought and behavior, headache, nausea and vomiting, delirium, and convulsions due to the osmotic swelling of the brain cells. If the water excess is only minimal, it is treated by restricting water intake. However, moderately severe hyponatremia impairs the kidney's ability to excrete the excess water, so a hypertonic saline solution (3 percent) may be given intravenously. If in addition to the low sodium level the plasma protein level is low, the administration of sodium will only result in edema. Thus plasma, salt-free albumin, or dextran needs to be given before attempting to correct the sodium deficit. Most surgeons avoid the syndrome by limiting intravenous fluids for the first 48 hr postoperatively and supplying adequate albumin and small amounts of sodium chloride daily.

HYPOKALEMIC METABOLIC ALKALOSIS

This is a development that may have serious results after open-heart surgery because it decreases myocardial contractility and thus decreases cardiac output [22]. The major causes of potassium depletion are:

1 Depletion of potassium preoperatively due to thiazide diuretics

2 Adrenal hyperactivity due to stress, which stimulates a potassium-sodium exchange system, resulting in increased reabsorption of sodium from the distal tubules of the kidney and a lowering of the plasma potassium

3 Osmotic diuresis from the administration of mannitol, urea, or other heavy solute loads, which results in more potassium being excreted

4 Poor myocardium, which increases the amount of potassium excreted

5 Hypothermia

6 In conjunction with hypochloremic alkalosis (alkalosis caused by a low chloride level). When there is a deficit of chloride ions for reabsorption along with sodium, sodium is excreted in the urine. Since a sodium deficiency cannot be tolerated, the normal mechanisms for conservation of sodium cause potassium and hydrogen ions to be exchanged for sodium in the distal tubule. If potassium ions are depleted, then hydrogen ions are excreted predominantly in exchange for sodium. This results in a depletion of the plasma hydrogen ions with an excess of bicarbonate ions and alkalosis. However, the urine becomes acid because of the increased secretion of the hydrogen ions. This phenomenon, termed paradoxical aciduria, was originally described by Van Slyke and Evans [90].

Signs and Symptoms

The signs and symptons of hypokalemic alkalosis are:

1 Acid urine (ph below 6) due to high hydrogen ion concentration with serum pH above 7.45.

2 Large amounts of potassium excreted in the urine—sometimes as high as 300 mEq/24 hr.

3 Cardiac arrhythmias and electrocardiograph changes that may or may not be present may show prolonged Q-T, compressed ST segment, decrease in T wave amplitude, with possible T wave inversion, and presence of U wave.

4 Anxiety, weakness, tremors, confusion, myoclonus, ileus, and seizures.

5 Serum potassium below 4 mEq/liter may or may not be present, since serum potassium does not always reflect total body potassium.

6 Signs of digitalis toxicity, since hypokalemia potentiates the action of digitalis. What has previously been a therapeutic level of digitalis may become toxic to the heart. Major signs of digitalis toxicity are atrial fibrillation or flutter with variable degrees of AV block and ventricular extrasystoles.

Treatment

Treatment is mainly directed toward prevention of severe alkalosis by replacing the daily loss of urinary potassium. Since a deficit of potassium is usually accompanied by a deficit of chloride, and to a lesser extent, a deficit of sodium, potassium chloride and sodium chloride are sometimes given [19]. The body homeostatic mechanisms selectively retain the chloride ions to replace the excess bicarbonate ions and retain the potassium ions to correct the potassium deficit. Studies made by Krohn demonstrated that patients lost the most potassium (up to 300 mEq in 24 hr) when less than 25 mEq of sodium in 24 hr was lost [91]. He found that in patients who lost less than 160 mEq of potassium in the urine in 24 hr, metabolic alkalosis could usually be prevented by replacing approximately 60 percent of the loss. When more than 160 mEq of potassium was lost, all the potassium had to be replaced to avoid or correct the alkalosis. Fifty percent dextrose in water with insulin was given with the high doses of potassium to drive the potassium into the cell and maintain the serum potassium concentration below 6 mEq per liter. As the patients improved, their potassium excretion decreased and the sodium excretion increased.

Some physicians feel that metabolic alkalosis can be prevented or lessened by the administration of a carbonic anhydrase inhibitor such as acetazolamide (Diamox), which causes hyperchloremia and a bicarbonate diuresis [29].

INFECTION

12

TYPES AND TREATMENT

The rate of infections after open-heart surgery is higher than in most surgical procedures because during surgery the heart and the great vessels are exposed to air for 2 to 5 hours. Antibiotics are routinely administered prophylactically following surgery. The major types of infection are endocarditis on a repaired valve or a prosthetic valve; mediastinitis following a sternal splitting incision; empyema in the pleural cavity, and, superficial wound infections.

In addition, the patient may develop an infection of the lungs, urinary tract, or a phlebitis. The presence of fever postoperatively cannot be used as a specific indication of an infection in patients who have been on cardiopulmonary bypass, since fever can be caused by many other things such as a reaction to the blood or certain drugs, or a metabolic response to stress. Fever during the first five days is expected, but if fever continues beyond the fifth day without any demonstrable cause (especially if the fever is higher than previously), subacute bacterial endocarditis is suspected. Serial and repeated blood cultures are necessary to establish the presence of endocarditis and the causative organism, since patients on antibiotics have been found to have as many as 14 negative cultures before one culture is positive [92].

Cytomegalic inclusion virus and post-pump virus syndrome can mimic bacterial endocarditis and make the diagnosis difficult without a positive blood culture. Cytomegalic inclusion virus produces symptoms similar to mononucleosis: fever, splenomegaly, lymphadenopathy, lymphocytosis, and abnormal lymphocytes. Post-pump virus syndrome is caused by a virus introduced into the patient. Incidence is higher when massive transfusions of blood are given.

Massive antibiotics are given if endocarditis is suspected. Best results are secured when the organism and its sensitivity are known and antibiotic therapy can be specific. When the patient's own valve is involved, the infection can be cured if intravenous antibiotics are continued for 10 to 12 weeks. If the involved valve is a prosthesis, it will act as a foreign body and the infection will not clear up. Reoperation and the insertion of a new valve will be necessary.

An osteomyelitis of the sternum is treated by removing all the wire sutures and leaving it open to drain. It may take 6 to 12 months to heal completely, but it will not heal unless the wires are removed. Some physicians believe zinc sulfate promotes wound healing.

NURSING INTERVENTION

The goal of nursing intervention is to prevent infection when possible, recognize any infection promptly, and institute proper management. Specific nursing measures are enumerated below.

- Observe, culture, and report any indication of infection preoperatively. Surgery should be postponed until an infection is cleared.
- Use careful suctioning procedure with a new catheter every time, sterile technique, and prevention of trauma to the mucosa.
- Maintain proper sterilization, packaging, and daily exchange of all oxygen therapy equipment.
- Use good aseptic techniques in the addition of all intravenous fluids and medications. All tubing and bottles should be changed every 24 or 48 hr.
- Maintain a closed system of chest drainage unless excessive drainage makes changing of bottles necessary.

- Maintain a closed system for urinary drainage using a bag with a bottom drain and a trap to prevent backflow (cystoflow). Any urine needed for culture should be withdrawn through the rubber catheter with a sterile needle and syringe.

- Give meticulous care to cutdown and other intravenous sites. If exposed to air, clean daily with half-strength hydrogen peroxide, rinse with saline, and dry. If a sterile dressing with antibiotic cream is used, the dressing should be changed daily and whenever soiled with drainage.

- Be diligent in maintaining patency and position of the endotracheal tube if patient is on the respirator and has a mediastinal incision, since a tracheostomy that has to be done before the fascia barrier has healed (usually five days) predisposes to a mediastinitis.

- Use care in the administration of antibiotics. Antibiotics are usually more effective when dissolved in a small amount of solute and given intravenously by buretrol. If the antibiotic is added to a liter

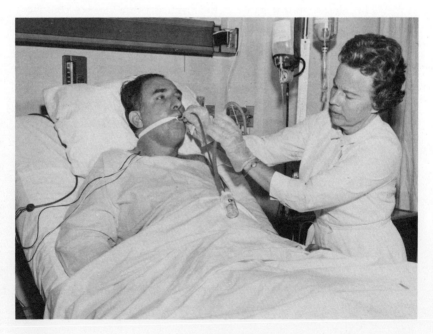

FIGURE 12–1   The use of a commercially available specimen trap that can be incorporated into the suction line makes obtaining a specimen from the endotracheal tube a quick process that minimizes contamination from other sources.

of intravenous fluid instead, any other drug added needs to be checked for compatibility or alteration of the pH of the fluid that may render the antibiotic ineffective.

- Culture any drainage from a wound promptly. Take a daily culture from the endotracheal tube or tracheostomy (Fig. 12-1), and culture the end of any Teflon or polyethylene tubing removed from a blood vessel.

- Instigate meticulous isolation technique when a positive culture report is received or when the character, amount, and odor of drainage from a wound makes the presence of infection highly suspected.

CARDIAC TAMPONADE

13

Cardiac tamponade is the term for an increase in the intrapericardial pressure caused by the collection of fluid or blood in the pericardial sac. It results in compression of the heart, limitation of diastolic filling, and decreased cardiac output. The most frequent cause in the postoperative open-heart surgery patient is bleeding from the myocardium. In most cases, the pericardium is left open and the mediastinal pleura is incised to allow for the drainage of blood via the chest tubes, thus lessening the danger of tamponade. However, in a study of 241 median sternotomy cases the creation of a pleural-pericardial communication for mediastinal drainage did not prevent tamponade from developing. A loculation of clot near the right atrium or superior vena cava effectively prevented venous return regardless of the open pericardium. The study also showed that late tamponade 8 to 30 days after operation occurred and was often misdiagnosed as cardiac failure or pulmonary embolism [93]. Causes of late tamponade are myocardial infarction after surgery, tubercular or viral pericarditis, and hemorrhage from anticoagulation.

SYMPTOMS

Symptoms are:

High central venous pressure (over 15 cm H_2O) with distension of jugular veins in the neck.

Left atrial pressure lower than right atrial pressure (CVP).

Decreased systolic blood pressure.

Narrowed pulse pressure (usually less than 15).

Pulse weak and thready.

Muffled heart sounds.

Paradoxical pulse, caused by the exaggerated effect of inspiration upon the blood pressure that results from the greater differential between intracardial pressure and pulmonary intravascular pressure. The blood pressure may fluctuate as much as 60 to 70 mm Hg during respiration. Occasionally it completely disappears during inspiration. To determine if a paradoxical pulse is present, use a blood pressure cuff to determine the pressure at which sounds are heard toward the end of expiration. Then slowly reduce the cuff pressure until the pressure is reached at which all systolic sounds are heard regardless of respiratory phase. If the difference is greater than 10 mm Hg, it is termed a paradoxical pulse.

Pericardial friction rub.

Apprehension and restlessness.

Decrease in EKG voltage since the blood in the pericardial sac "insulates" the myocardium from the EKG electrode.

TREATMENT

The aim of the treatment is to remove the fluid that is causing cardiac compression. Usually needle aspiration (pericardicentesis) of the fluid is attempted first with a large caliber needle (16 to 20 gauge) at the apex (1 cm below and 1 cm to the left of the xiphoid process). If the aspirating needle is attached to an EKG machine as a sterile electrode, the electrical tracing may be helpful in determining the position of the needle tip, for when the needle touches the ventricle, the current indicates the injury by an elevation of the ST segment. One indication that the blood is from the pericardial sac is that it will not usually clot. Usually aspiration is sufficient, but when repeated aspirations are necessary, a thoractomy is usually done with the formation of a pericardial window to obtain permanent pericardial drainage.

RENAL FAILURE

14

The kidneys are responsible for the conversion of waste products of cellular metabolism into urine that is then eliminated from the body. By selectively eliminating certain electrolytes with fluid and reabsorption of approximately 80 percent of the water, the normal kidney maintains the fluid and electrolyte balance in the body. A decrease in the effectiveness of the kidneys to excrete a normal amount of urine has been termed oliguria or renal insufficiency. If no urine is excreted, it is referred to as anuria, or renal failure. Some physicians use the term renal failure to denote a daily urine output of less than 400 ml. Postoperative open-heart surgery patients are monitored hourly for urine volume, specific gravity, and pH. If the urine output drops to 15 ml in one hour, and does not recover the second hour, it is a cause for concern. Since low output can be due to a mechanical obstruction of the Foley catheter (plug, kink, and so on) this possibility should always be investigated.

CAUSES OF RENAL FAILURE

The development of renal failure in patients who have not previously had kidney damage usually results from:

1 Cardiovascular insufficiency, with a blood pressure below 70 systolic and severe vasoconstriction.

2 Volume deficiency due to inadequate volume replacement at time of surgery, or severe preoperative dehydration from use of diuretics and limitation of sodium intake.

3 Kidney deficiency or acute tubular necrosis, which may result from ischemia from any of the above or be caused by:

(a) Allergic reaction to incompatible blood.

(b) Luminal occlusion of renal tubules caused by hemolysis of red cells after bypass procedure, with precipitation of hemoglobin.

(c) Lack of adequate blood flow during bypass period or prolonged bypass.

(d) Emboli to renal arteries, which may be bilateral.

To differentiate in the early stages between renal failure due to primary damage to the kidney and that due to inadequate renal perfusion because of volume deficiency, the following table of diagnostic clues is helpful, although individual differences exist among patients:

Primary Kidney Damage	Inadequate Renal Perfusion (Prerenal failure)
Normal or elevated central venous pressure	Low central venous pressure
Rising serum creatinine and BUN	BUN concentration rising proportionately higher than creatinine
Urine to plasma creatinine concentration ratio less than 20 mEq/l	Urine to plasma creatinine concentration ratio greater than 20 mEq/l
Urine specific gravity from 1.010–1.014	Urine with high specific gravity (may be as high as 1.035)
Urinary sodium concentration of 30–40 mEq/l	Urinary sodium concentration less than 20 mEq/l
Urine to plasma osmolality ratio less than 1.5	Urine to plasma osmolality ratio greater than 1.5 [94]

Sometimes a mannitol test is used to determine the cause of the oliguria. Twelve and a half to 25 gm of mannitol is given intravenously over a period of 10 min. Each 12.5 gm of mannitol should result in the excretion of approximately 125 ml urine if the oliguria is caused by volume deficiency. Since the proportion of water excreted is greater than the sodium excreted, a preexisting elevated level of sodium will be increased. Also, if mannitol is not excreted, it remains primarily within the intravascular space and may contribute to the development of heart failure. Thus many physicians prefer to use the method of rapid administration (within 30 min) of 500 cc of a balanced solution such as Ringer's lactate while observing the response of the CVP and urine output. An increase in the CVP indicates cardiac decompensation, an increase in urine output indicates volume deficiency, and no increase (or very little increase) in urine output indicates kidney damage.

Management of the patient with prerenal failure is based on prompt treatment of the underlying cause, to avoid kidney damage that may result from ischemia or precipitation of hemoglobin in the tubules. Vasodilator drugs may be given to increase the blood supply to the kidney. Diuretics such as Furosemide or Ethacrynic acid are frequently given to stimulate urine output to "flush out" any hemoglobin. Some physicians prefer to give osmotic diuretics like mannitol.

If kidney damage has occurred, the treatment is directed toward maintaining as normal a balance of fluid and electrolytes as possible so the kidney will have time to heal and renal function can be restored. The oliguric phase may last several days to three weeks, averaging 10 to 12 days. If renal function was adequate preoperatively, the recovery rate is better than 50 percent [95].

TREATMENT

The main aspects of the treatment include:

- *Careful monitoring of fluid intake.* Intravenous fluids are given to replace the insensible loss from respiration (500 ml) and skin (500 ml) plus replacement volume for volume of any urine put out. Although replacement of other than urinary loss would usually mean an intake of 1000 ml, many physicians prefer to limit the total to 400 ml, plus urinary loss to avoid a circulatory overload. If the patient is on a diet, the amount of water derived from the metabolism of food must be included in the intake total. Fever can cause loss of more water, so intake needs to be increased for fever. Zimmerman believes the fluid requirements are increased 10 percent for each degree of fever [19].

- *Daily weights* to determine excess or deficient fluid administration. A patient on only intravenous fluids can be expected to lose 0.5 to 1.0 lb daily. For every 2.2 lb (1 kg) gained, the patient is storing 1 liter of fluid.

- *Maintenance of serum potassium* within normal limits, to prevent cardiac arrest due to hyperkalemia. Serial EKGs are used as well as serum electrolyte studies to determine the presence of potassium intoxication. Hypertonic glucose and insulin are sometimes used to drive the potassium into the cells. Hypertonic sodium bicarbonate is sometimes preferred for potassium toxicity. Cation-exchange resins (usually given rectally) may be given to remove excess potassium. If hypocalcemia is present, calcium gluconate is usually given since it antagonizes potassium. Since some penicillins contain potassium, this content should be taken into consideration.

- *Restricting water intake* for hyponatremia rather than giving sodium. Sodium bicarbonate may be given for severe acidosis.

- *Prevention of infection* by use of a closed system for urinary drainage, care of intravenous entry sites, aseptic techniques for wound and other incisions, and good pulmonary management. Antibiotics are generally used, but Garamycin, Colistin, Polymixin, and Kanamycin, which are toxic to the kidney, are usually avoided.

- *Provision of adequate calories* to prevent negative nitrogen balance with resultant metabolic acidosis. Nonessential proteins are not given. Parenteral hyperalimentation has already been discussed under fluids and electrolytes. Calories are usually provided by hypertonic glucose and amino acids intravenously, with oral intake of butter and hard candies. Sometimes a few ice chips made from freezing 50 percent glucose are allowed.

- *Use of anabolic steroids* like testosterone or methandrostenolone to stimulate anabolic activity and decrease protein breakdown.

- *Use of only fresh blood* when transfusion is necessary, since bank blood has a higher level of potassium and the red cell survival rate is shorter. Transfusions are usually given only for hematocrits below 22 unless other symptoms of need for blood are present.

- *Adjustment of dosage of drugs* that are excreted by the kidney since the toxic level of the drug can be reached with a smaller dose and the effects are more prolonged. Short-acting preparations of digitalis and barbiturates should be given, with a preference for drugs that are metabolized primarily by the liver.

- *Restriction of magnesium intake* both in IV fluids and in antacid therapy. Most antacids have a high magnesium and sodium content. If antacids are indicated, aluminum hydroxide is usually given.

- *Encouragement to ambulation and oral intake* as soon as possible.

- *Use of lemon juice and glycerine swabs* to keep the pH of the mouth acid and thereby prevent stomatitis.

- *Prophylactic dialysis* is usually indicated for a BUN above 100 mg percent, hyperkalemia of 6.5 to 7 mEq/liter, or blood pH below 7.2. Some physicians prefer to wait rather than dialyze before uremic problems occur. Hemodialysis is usually the method of choice, but for the patient with precarious cardiac status, peritoneal dialysis may be preferred.

- *Careful monitoring* needs to be continued when the patient begins to diurese. Although the output may be as much as 6 liters per day, sodium and potassium imbalances as well as acidosis may complicate recovery.

PAIN

15

PATIENT'S RESPONSE TO PAIN

Although postoperative pain is accepted by the surgeons and nurses as unavoidable and natural, the patient may feel that pain is the most difficult aspect of his postoperative period. The experience of pain encompasses the stimulus of pain, the perception of pain, and the reaction to pain. The stimulus to a pain receptor is carried to the central nervous system. The perception of pain is localized in the thalamus and is interpreted in the cerebral cortex. Once pain has been perceived in the thalamus, the stimulus moves in circular patterns and sets off reverberating pain circuits in the cerebral cortex that intensify all the patient's reactions to pain. His reactions to pain may include autonomic, skeletal muscle, and psychic reactions [96], examples of which are:

Autonomic reactions
Alterations in blood pressure, with severe deep pain resulting in hypotension

Inhibition of peristalsis because of increased secretion of epinephrine

Shift of blood to heart and lungs with resultant pallor

Tachypnea, tachycardia

Increased perspiration

Skeletal muscle reactions (Fig. 15–1)

Clenched fists

Grimacing, clenching of teeth, tight lips, frowns, wrinkles in the forehead

Gripping of chest with hands

Restless purposeless movements of extremities

Muscle rigidity and spasm

Psychic reactions

Moaning, groaning, or crying

Negativism

Irritability

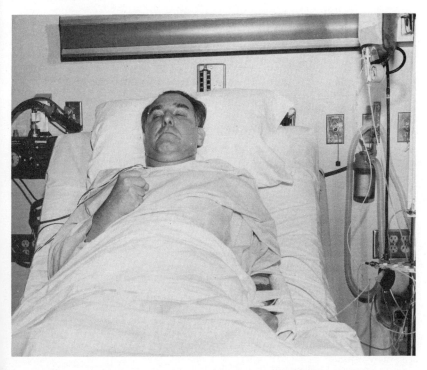

FIGURE 15–1   A patient's posture, tension, and rigidity may be indicators of pain.

Anxiety

Attention focused on self, with lessening of response to environment

Use of various adaptive mechanisms

Variables that Influence Patient's Response to Pain

The experience of pain is subjective and differs markedly from one patient to another because it is influenced by many physiological, cultural, and psychological variables. These variables must be assessed and correlated with the reactions to pain the patient is exhibiting to provide a basis for successful nursing intervention.

1 *Physiological variables* include the location, intensity, and duration of the pain. Pain that is present over a long period of time reduces the capacity of the patient to tolerate pain. Discomforts occurring in other areas of the body at the same time tend to heighten a patient's perception of pain.

2 *Cultural conditioning* influences what the individual regards as painful and how he reacts to pain. Some persons feel that pain is just recompense for wrong-doing and that it should be borne bravely for the spiritual gains that are derived. Women are usually encouraged to express pain more freely than men, since stoicism is sometimes equated with manliness, and loss of control is considered undesirable.

3 *Psychological factors* have been associated with the reaction to pain rather than the sensation of pain and thus they involve the higher cognitive processes [97].

Variables that Affect the Patient's Perception of Pain

Variables that may increase or decrease the perception of pain are:

1 *Previous pain experiences,* since the patient usually tends to transfer the knowledge gained from past experiences with pain to new situations.

2 *Characteristic manner* of perceiving and interpreting pain. Petrie and Wolk found that people interpreted pain in one of three ways ([98]):

(a) *Reducers.* These people tend subjectively to decrease what they feel. They are tolerant of suffering with pain and of bombardment with sensation, and intolerant of the stress of monotony and isolation.

(b) *Augmenters.* This is the opposite of the reducers. These persons tend subjectively to magnify their feelings. They are intolerant of suffering from pain, but tolerant of monotony and isolation.

(c) *Moderates.* Moderates are persons who do not appreciably alter what they feel. They are moderately tolerant of suffering from pain and also of monotony and isolation.

3 *Adaptive mechanisms,* such as intellectualization, withdrawal, and denial, help the patient handle pain with a minimum of physical and mental discomfort [99].

4 *Presence of anxiety,* which tends to lower the threshold of pain because anxiety as well as pain activates the thalamo-cortical circuit and thus the cerebral cortex is in an excitable state that augments pain perception [100].

5 *Association of pain with threat to life,* especially when the patient experiences sudden severe pain when he previously was relatively free from pain.

6 *Depth of knowledge and understanding* of the cause and implication of the pain.

7 *Presence, attitudes, and suggestions* of family and professional staff. They influence a patient's experience of pain and his manner of responding to the pain.

NURSING INTERVENTION

After the response and the influencing variables have been identified, a nursing plan for intervention to interrupt or modify the pain in the circuit from pain source to pain reaction can be initiated and implemented. Such a plan usually includes measures to alleviate pain at its source, alleviate the perception of pain in the thalmus, and alleviate the reaction to pain in the cerebral cortex.

Measures to Alleviate Pain at Its Source

- Better support of the endotracheal tube.
- Use of a nasogastric tube for abdominal distension.
- Prevention of any pull on chest tubes.

- Frequent changes of position with several persons working together and synchronizing their efforts, and maintenance of good anatomical alignment for the patient with support as needed to prevent muscle strain.

- Use of a pillow to support the chest wound when a patient coughs.

- Meticulous care of mouth and lips to prevent cracking and sores.

- Use of anesthetic lozenges, viscous xylocaine, or warm saline gargles to relieve throat soreness after patient is extubated.

- Assisting the physician to instill small amounts of xylocaine down the endotracheal tube or to infiltrate locally an exceptionally sensitive nerve at the site of insertion of the chest tube.

- Maintenance of cleanliness of skin, dressings, and bed linen to reduce discomfort as much as possible.

Measures to Reduce the Central Perception of Pain

- *Analgesics* that increase the threshold of pain in the thalamus. Small doses (3–5 mg) of morphine intravenously is usually the preferred drug when the patient is on the respirator. Morphine both allays apprehension and lessens the perception of pain. If the patient is not on a respirator, other analgesics are usually given which do not have such a depressant effect on respirations. If Innovar has been used for the anesthetic, any narcotic given within 6 to 8 hr after surgery should be reduced to one-third the usual dose because of the potentiating effect of Innovar on a narcotic.

- *Tranquilizers* given with analgesics increase the effectiveness of the analgesic by altering the mood of the patient.

- *Autosuggestion* or telling the patient the drug will help him usually adds to the effectiveness of any medication.

- *Distraction* or redirecting the patient's attention from the pain to something more pleasant such as music or conversation may decrease the perception of pain.

- *Identification* of any factors as anxiety or tension that might inhibit the action of the drug.

- *Administration of medication* when patient exhibits signs of having pain instead of withholding medication until patient asks for it, since if pain has become severe, it will be intensified by the increased cerebral cortex excitability.

- *The use of low concentrations of inhalational anesthetics* such as nitrous oxide or trichloroethylene postoperatively, especially prior to coughing and deep breathing, has been recommended by some physicians [101].

Measures to Reduce the Reaction to Pain

- *Preoperative psychologic conditioning,* which has been termed the most important single factor in postoperative response [101]. If the patient has been told to expect some pain, what causes the pain, and that he will be given some medication to reduce the pain, he will usually have fewer complaints of pain. Janis found that many patients defended themselves against their disturbing fantasies about surgery by denying the likelihood that they would have any pain postoperatively. When this illusion was shattered, they reacted with anger, resentment, and intolerance to the pain [102].

- *Allowing patient to have more control* over deciding what to do for pain. Studies have shown that the way a nurse interacts with a patient can significantly affect his attitude and response to pain [103]. When patients were encouraged by a nurse they trusted to participate in deciding what method of relief would be used for their pain, they experienced greater relief from their pain.

- *Remaining with the patient who is having a painful experience.* This helps to reduce the anxiety and the feeling of isolation that intensify the pain experience. A family member may be allowed to stay with the patient if the presence is beneficial to the patient. The family member's contribution is usually greater when they receive some instruction from the nurse on therapeutic behavior and when they are recognized for their contribution.

- *The use of such expressive actions* as touching and listening to the patient to establish a relationship that helps to meet the needs for dependency, love, and self-esteem, since such inter-personal relationships may raise the pain reaction threshold.

- *Allowing time for mobilization of defense mechanisms.* Before a painful procedure is started, tell the patient what is going to be done and how he can expect to feel, which allows him a little time to mobilize his adaptive defense mechanisms, unless it has been found that the patient is unable to mobilize his defenses constructively. Giving pain medication before a painful procedure generally decreases pain perception in the thalamus as well as decreasing the reaction to pain in the cerebral cortex.

In a few instances, the experience of pain may be prolonged and exaggerated by the emotional needs of the patient. This patient is motivated, often unconsciously, to tolerate the pain in order to secure certain "secondary gains" [104].

Some secondary gains are control of the actions of others, avoidance of responsibility, avoidance of criticism, and allowance of dependency. Preoperative conditioning and a plan of postoperative care that satisfies the emotional needs of the patient will usually prevent him from using pain to express his anger, ease his anxiety, or for secondary gain. The patient with limited emotional resources to meet the stresses of the operation may cling to pain as a coping device and as a means to manipulate his environment. He needs emotional support and reassurance from the staff and needs to be consistently encouraged to talk about the other things that are bothering him (such as his feelings of inadequacy, family, and interpersonal relationships) and work to solve any underlying problem situations [100].

After the nurse has implemented her plan for the relief of pain, the results need to be evaluated and the intervention modified as indicated. To provide for continuity of care of the patient she needs to record successful intervention on the nursing care plan.

ABNORMAL HEART RHYTHMS
AND PACEMAKERS

16

Abnormal heart rhythms need to be carefully observed by the nurse. Any change in the basic rhythm should especially be noted and an EKG strip saved for the record. (In another section, specific drugs for abnormal heart rhythms are discussed.) In addition to drugs, an artificial electrical pacemaker may be indicated to stimulate ventricular contraction in the following conditions:

- *Complete block of the AV node* (also referred to as third-degree block), which may be followed by the ventricle taking over the pacing function at a slow rate. If the ventricular rate is less than 40 or 45 beats per minute, the cardiac output may be insufficient to support consciousness or adequate coronary, cerebral, and renal perfusion. Since the transition from supraventricular to ventricular pacing may be sudden and accompanied by loss of consciousness and convulsions, and it is difficult to place a transvenous pacemaker in an actively convulsing patient, an electrode catheter may be placed when the patient develops second-degree block. Heart block, which may develop following open-heart surgery, is generally caused by digitalis toxicity or sutures placed in the bundle of His in the process of repairing an intra-atrial septal defect or ventricular septal defect or inserting a prosthetic valve.

- *Bradycardia* that does not respond to drugs, since the heart is most efficient at a rate of 80 to 100.
- *Atrial fibrillation or flutter* with a slow ventricular response. This may predispose to ventricular tachyarrhythmias.
- *Abnormal heart rhythms* that are life-threatening and unresponsive to medical therapy.
- *Cardiac standstill.*

The electrocardiograph of a patient with a pacemaker shows an artifact preceding each QRS that is initiated by the pacemaker. The artifact is sometimes referred to as a "blip" or a "spike." The amplitude of the blip on the EKG is an indication of the electrical power that is reaching the ventricular wall since two blocks equals 10 mv. When the catheter is in the ventricle, the impulse is conducted in a retrograde manner and the ventricle depolarizes as though there was an ectopic focus. Since the catheter is in the right ventricle, the right side of the ventricle depolarizes before the left side and the EKG resembles a ventricular rhythm with a left bundle branch block. If the catheter moves, the origin of the impulse will change and the complex will appear different. The artifact is larger in the pacemakers termed unipolar than in those termed bipolar.

TYPES OF PACEMAKERS

There are four major types of artificial pacemakers: fixed-rate, demand, atrial synchronous, and paired.

Fixed-rate

These pacemakers deliver an electrical impulse for contraction to the ventricle at a regular rate that is predetermined. The main disadvantages of this type of pacemaker are that it limits the circulation by 25 or 30 percent since the ventricular contraction has no relationship to the atrial contraction (which fills the ventricle with blood) and may occur when there is very little blood in the ventricle; and it may compete with the patient's own pacemaker, and an electrical stimulus for contraction may be delivered during the vulnerable period of repolarization and set off a ventricular tachycardia and/or fibrillation. Although the incidence of death produced by pacemaker competition is unknown, in one group of patients the death rate was five times greater with fixed-rate pacemakers [105].

Demand

Demand pacemakers are considered much safer than fixed-rate pacemakers because they do not compete with the patient's own pacemaker. If the patient has a P wave followed by a QRS complex within the preset period of time, the pacemaker gives no electrical stimulation. However, if the QRS does not follow within the time period, then the pacer gives a stimulus that initiates prompt ventricular depolarization.

Atrial Synchronous

These pacemakers take advantage of atrial transport by picking up the P wave from the SA node, amplifying it electronically, and then transmitting it to an electrode implanted in the ventricular wall that initiates ventricular depolarization (for example, the Atricor). The contraction of the atria gives 25 percent more blood to the heart than the fixed-rate pacer. In the event of failure of the SA node, the pacemaker contains a fixed-rate circuit that automatically assumes control of the heartbeat. The disadvantage of this type of pacer is that it requires a thoracotomy for its installation and in a majority of cases, batteries last a little less than two years. The pacemaker contains three wires, one of which is sewn on the atrium and the other two are sewn on the ventricle (one serves as an auxiliary electrode). The Atricor contains a built-in blocking system to prevent ventricular tachycardia. When the atrial rate exceeds 120, a 2:1 block starts and only every other impulse will be transmitted to the electrode in the ventricle. If the atrial rate exceeds 180 per minute, the block becomes 3:1. When the atrial rate slows below 120, every S-A impulse is again transmitted to the electrode in the ventricle and every P wave is again followed by a QRS. The EKG for an Atricor shows a P wave with a constant interval before every blip, with the blip followed immediately by the QRS.

Paired

Paired or coupled pacing has been used experimentally in patients with tachycardia and those with low myocardial contractile force. The second pacing stimulus is timed to fall immediately after the termination of the absolute refractory period, and causes an electrical systole without a mechanical systole. The electrical systole is followed by a second refractory period, so the refractory period during which the heart is unresponsive to other electrical stimuli is essentially doubled. The prolongation of refractiveness slows the heart rate. Another consequence of paired electrical stimulation is augmentation of the myocardial contractile force. This is believed to represent a sustained form of postextrasystolic potentiation. The danger of paired pacing is that the second impulse is delivered very close to the vulnerable period, and ventricular fibrillation could be the result [106,29].

METHODS OF ARTIFICIALLY PACING THE HEART

External Pacemakers on the Chest Wall

These pacemakers use two electrodes on the anterior chest (one at the apex and the other at the base of the heart) to deliver an electrical stimulus that will cause the heart to contract. Electrode paste is applied to the skin under the electrodes and they are secured with a rubber strap fastened about the chest. The electrodes are connected to a fixed-rate pacemaker machine and the rate is set for the desired number of electrical stimulations for heart contractions per minute. This is extremely uncomfortable for a conscious patient, since a high voltage is necessary to pace the heart through the chest wall. It is also rarely effective in cases of cardiac standstill.

Percutaneous Pacing

Percutaneous pacing is the emergency method of artificially pacing the heart; it has almost supplanted the use of the external electrodes. This procedure may use two thin, insulated Elgiloy wires prethreaded through a long 20- or 21-gauge thin wall needle and bent back about one-eighth of an inch at the point. The needle is introduced percutaneously into the right ventricle and withdrawn gently, leaving the two wires affixed in the ventricle [107]. The two wires are then connected to the terminals of the cable from the pacer machine and the machine is activated. Either a fixed-rate or a demand pacer machine can be used. If the two wires are touching within the ventricle, current will not flow. It is necessary to insert another wire beneath the skin and connect it to the positive terminal. Both heart wires can be connected to the negative terminal.

Also available for percutaneous pacing are commercial pacing probes such as the Elecath. These probes utilize a needle with a removable stylet. The bipolar probe is inserted after the stylet is removed and has a natural curve that facilitates its contact with the myocardium. After the needle is withdrawn, the pacer probe is connected to the pacemaker by a special connector apparatus.

During the surgical process, temporary electrode wires are sometimes placed in the myocardium and brought out through the lower end of the incision. They are then connected to a pacemaker as described in percutaneous pacing.

Transvenous Pacing

Transvenous pacing with an external pacemaker is the temporary method of choice for pacing the heart when there is adequate time to pass the catheter into the right ventricle via a major vein. Most physicians think that the catheter is more easily passed into the heart when it is inserted into the vein of the left arm. The saphenous, basilic, subclavian, or jugular vein may be used, although the jugular is usually reserved for an implanted pacer. The catheter is either passed under fluoroscopy or by the use of the electrocardiogram obtained from within the heart, using the catheter as an exploring electrode. The fluoroscopic method has the advantage that the catheter's course can be visualized during the procedure and thus it gives the operator better control over its position. However, emergency conditions may not allow time for fluoroscopy, and the use of the electrocardiogram is indicated.

When the EKG is used, the proximal end of the pacemaker catheter is attached to the chest lead terminal of the EKG machine. The EKG tracing will show the position of the catheter tip as it advances through the heart chambers. When the tip of the catheter enters the atrium, the tracing will show a large and inverted P wave. At the midatrial level the P wave will become diphasic. When the catheter enters the right ventricle, the P wave will become small and positive while the ventricular complex will increase in size, the ST segment will become elevated, and the T wave will become inverted [108].

Whatever method is used for placement, the best results are obtained when the catheter is wedged between the trabeculae carneae and the ventricle wall (Fig. 16–1). The catheter is then connected to either a fixed-rate or demand pacer. The demand pacer is usually preferred in order to avoid the dangers associated with competitive pacing.

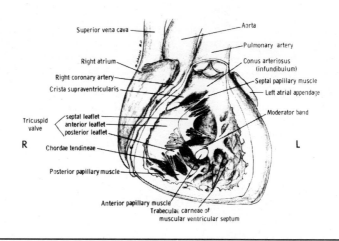

FIGURE 16-1 Schematic frontal view of the heart with the anterior right ventricular wall removed. A transvenous pacemaker is usually wedged between the chordae tendineae and the trabecular carni of the right ventricle. *(From M. E. Silverman and R. C. Schlant, Functional Anatomy of the Cardiovascular System, in J. W. Hurst and R. B. Logue (eds), "The Heart," McGraw-Hill Book Company, New York, 1970. Used by permission.)*

When the electrode has been passed via a vein in the arm, the arm is usually immobilized for 2 or 3 days because the tip of the catheter is easily displaced. The patient is also instructed not to sleep on his right side for a few days because the catheter is more apt to perforate in this position. The insertion of the catheter is watched closely for any signs of infection such as redness or swelling. External pacemakers have a control to adjust the rate and the intensity of the electrical stimulus (voltage) (Fig. 16-2).

Implanted Transvenous Pacemakers

These pacemakers are used in patients who need a pacemaker beyond a few days but who are not good candidates for epicardial implants that require a thoracotomy. Demand pacers are nearly always used. The battery lasts two to three years and then the pacemaker module needs to be replaced. The transvenous electrode is usually passed via the external jugular vein with subpectoral implantation of the power module. Although the electrode is usually placed in the ventricle as it is for temporary transvenous pacing, some physicians are suggesting the use of atrial pacing in intermittent sinus arrest and marked sinus

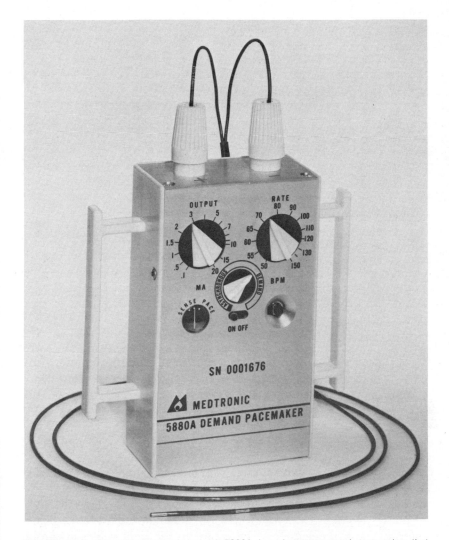

FIGURE 16–2   The new Medtronic model 5880A is a battery-powered pacemaker that operates in either the demand or fixed-rate mode. It incorporates filtering circuitry that block the ac leakage currents and built-in shielding to prevent most electrical interference. If interference is stronger than 100 mV, the pacemaker output is suppressed. *(Photograph courtesy of Medtronic, Inc., Minneapolis, Minn.)*

bradycardia [105]. For atrial pacing, the electrode wires are placed near the junction of the superior vena cava and the right atrium.

Furmin [109] has given the following suggestions to decrease the incidence of problems with implanted transvenous pacemakers:

1 To reduce electrical malfunctioning, the guide wire should be inserted and removed gently so the helical springs are not damaged. The guide wire should not be left in the patient after the catheter is implanted.

2 To avoid skin erosion over the pulse generator an adequate pouch should be developed at the time of implantation, and adequate drainage provided to evacuate the blood and serum from beneath the skin flap.

3 To avoid loosening of the fixation ligatures at the point of insertion, mersilene ligature should be used instead of silk, as silk loses tensile strength.

4 To prevent a recoil movement that may result in their returning to the right atrium, catheters should be inserted without any slack.

5 To prevent outputs below the myocardial threshold, pulse generators should be set at maximum when implanted.

Implanted Transthoracic Pacemakers

These are used in patients who are relatively young (especially when the ventricle is diseased) because they can tolerate the thoracotomy and they need the advantage of being able to increase their heart rate with exercise. Although fixed-rate pacers can be implanted, the practice is to use atrial synchronous pacers only.

Parasternal Mediastinotomy

Parasternal mediastinotomy is a new approach to implanted epicardial leads; it avoids the risk of a formal thoracotomy procedure and also eliminates the problems of migration, malposition, and instability of the transvenous catheter electrodes. Adequate exposure for placement of the two electrodes 1 cm apart on the right ventricle can be obtained by resection of only the fourth, fifth, and sixth costal cartilages. Since this procedure can be done under local anesthesia with little discomfort postoperatively, it may become the preferred method for implanted pacemaker leads [110].

Radiofrequency Pacemakers

These pacemakers, developed at Yale University, eliminate the need for wire electrodes. A tiny receiver is implanted beneath the pericardium and a transmitter worn outside the body transmits radio energy that is converted by the receiver to electrical pacing stimuli, which is then delivered to the ventricles by platinum disk electrodes [111].

Piezoelectric Pacemakers

These pacemakers, which require no batteries, are in the experimental development stage. These devices convert the mechanical energy derived from the contraction of the ventricle into electricity which is then used to deliver pacing stimuli to the heart [111].

Radio-activated Isotope Pacemakers

Using an isotope of plutonium, the pacemaker could be implanted and last 10 years or more. It is currently under investigation by the Atomic Energy Commission [111].

PACEMAKER FUNCTION

Implanted pacemakers may have a fixed voltage (usually 11.2 milliamperes), but in most models the rate can be adjusted either before or after implantation by means of a surgical skin needle inserted in the rate control. When the electrical impulse given by the pacemaker is immediately followed by a QRS (depolarization of the ventricle), the pacemaker is said to "capture" the ventricle (Fig. 16–3). When the impulse does not capture the ventricle or when there is intermittent capture, it is probably caused by:

1 High myocardial threshold, which is probably the result of edema around the electrode wires

2 Broken electrode wire, which usually gives no problem lying flat, but will cause difficulty in the upright position

3 Weak batteries in the pacemaker module

4 Electrode has become dislodged from the ventricular wall and hangs loose, making intermittent contact with the myocardium when the position is changed

5 Electrode has perforated the myocardium, which may be accompanied by precordial pain or muscular contraction of the diaphragm or upper abdominal muscles

6 Insulation leak in the electrode wire

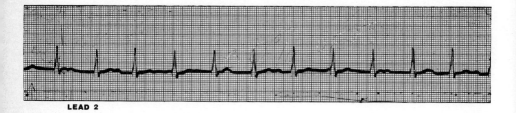

LEAD 2

MCL₁

FIGURE 16–3   EKG tracings from lead 2 and *MCL₁* that demonstrate a pacemaker capture rhythm. Since the rhythm originates in the right ventricle, it looks like a right ventricular rhythm. The pacemaker blip can be seen immediately preceding each *QRS*.

An EKG and chest x-rays that include lateral views will help in the diagnosis of pacemaker malfunction. If the EKG shows no artifact, a small radio (tuned to a location where no station is heard) can be held to the skin adjacent to the implanted module. A definite "click" on the radio that corresponds to the rate of the pacemaker indicates that the problem is caused by a high threshold, broken electrode wire, or weak batteries. If no audible click is heard, the problem is probably a defect in the circuit or battery failure [112]. Battery failure is also detected sometimes by a change in the wave form of the pacemaker stimulus; this change can be demonstrated with a "stopper" oscilloscope [113].

CARE OF PATIENTS WITH PACEMAKERS

The management of patients with pacemakers includes the following medical and nursing responsibilities:

- Close observation of the EKG for any malfunction of the pacemaker.

- The use of lidocaine or other myocardial depressants to control the frequent premature beats that may occur in the first few days.

- The use of heparin for 3–5 days. Most physicians feel that there is no danger of clots forming around the electode after 5 days.

- Disconnecting an external pacemaker before defibrillation. When a patient with an implanted pacemaker module needs to be defibrillated, the paddles should be placed perpendicular to the wires.

- Careful protection and insulation of pacemaker wires left in the heart that come out through the chest wall from contact with any other electrical appliance.

- Proper grounding of any pacemaker that operates on wall current to prevent one piece of electrical equipment from developing a potential higher than another machine in relation to the common ground potential, since electrical current can then flow through the patient and induce ventricular fibrillation. The exclusive use of battery-powered machines is recommended by some physicians.

- Meticulous care of the skin around the insertion site to prevent infection. Once infection develops around a prosthetic device, the device has to be removed. If the infection extends to the electrode, a thoracotomy will be necessary since an electrode that has been in place for a period of time cannot be pulled back out without risking tearing of the myocardium.

- Proper repositioning of an electrode that has perforated the myocardium or become displaced.

- Increasing the voltage on an external pacemaker until the pacemaker "captures" the ventricle.

- The use of medical measures to lower the myocardial threshold when a high threshold is the reason the pacemaker does not capture the ventricle. Measures suggested by Dr. Walker [114] are: (1) Elevation of serum potassium. Potassium should be given without glucose or insulin. (2) Administration of glucocorticoids. (3) Sympathetic stimulation, which may be done by the administration of epinephrine, norepinephrine, and sometimes Isuprel. (4) Exercise, and (5) Lowering serum calcium.

- Periodic testing of a demand pacemaker whose impulse is being suppressed because the patient's own heart rate is faster than the pacemaker rate. All demand pacemakers have a magnetic switch so a magnet can be placed over the pacemaker to cut out the demand mode so the pacemaker will pace at a fixed rate. Thus any problem with the pacemaker can be identified and corrected.

17

Any patient who is receiving digitalis (or received digitalis in the immediate preoperative period) should be observed for signs of digitalis toxicity. The incidence of toxicity is higher in patients with severely damaged myocardium and hypokalemia. The normal half-life of digitalis is 30 to 38 hr. In renal failure the half-life extends to 82 hr. The use of the heart bypass pump or dialysis has very little effect on the level of digitalis. It should be remembered that anything that stimulates the vagus (as for example the Valsalva maneuver) has an enhanced effect when digitalis toxicity is present.

SYMPTOMS

Manifestations of toxicity are evidenced in the gastrointestinal system, neuro-ophthalmogical system, and cardiovascular system.

Gastrointestinal symptons
Anorexia, nausea and vomiting
Diarrhea

Neuro-ophthalmological symptoms
Headache and restlessness
Mood changes and irritability
Visual disturbances such as colored vision and photophobia
Convulsions, stupor, and coma (rare)

Cardiovascular symptoms
Changes in the rhythm due to the increased cardiac irritability evidenced by:
Premature ventricular contractions which frequently occur coupled with the sinus or supraventricular contraction (bigeminy)
Atrial tachycardia
Nodal tachycardia
Ventricular tachycardia which may progress to ventricular fibrillation.
Changes in the method of conduction in the AV node which may result in first, second, or third degree AV block with AV dissociation

TREATMENT

Treatment of mild digitalis toxicity may require no more specific therapy than withdrawing the digitalis. For life-threatening extrasystoles, the usual management includes:

- Discontinuance of the drug.

- Administration of potassium. 20 mEq KCl is usually added to 250 to 500 ml of intravenous fluid and given over a period of 1 to 2 hr while the EKG is continuously monitored. Potassium is contraindicated in the presence of complete heart block because it may further impair conduction and result in more serious arrhythmias.

- Withholding of diuretics that result in urinary excretion of potassium and intravenous infusions of concentrated carbohydrates (higher than 5 percent) that drive potassium into the cell.

- Use of EDTA (ethylene-diamine-tetra-acetate) to bind the serum calcium, since calcium potentiates the effect of digitalis on cardiac irritability and conduction. EDTA, 600 mg to 1 gm is added to 250 ml of intravenous fluid and given IV over 30 to 60 min. Results have not proven consistently beneficial and administration may result in renal damage, so the value of EDTA is controversial.

- Placement of a transvenous pacer for stand-by use in the development of complete heart block, when the patient does not already have a pacer in place.

- Administration of myocardial depressant drugs for ventricular extrasystoles or ventricular tachycardia: *Propranolol hydrochloride* (Inderal) is the usual myocardial depressant drug of choice when digitalis toxicity is present. One to five milligrams may be given by a slow intravenous push at a rate that does not exceed 1 mg/min. Oral administration is preferred, with 10 to 30 mg given four times a day. Since the drug blocks the action of catecholamines on the heart, it is usually not given if the patient is in cardiogenic shock. *Diphenylhydantoin* (Dilantin) is sometimes used if hypotension is present, as it is effective in suppressing ventricular irritability that is digitalis-induced. Dosage is 250 mg given by a slow intravenous push, or 200 to 600 mg orally a day in divided doses may be given. *Pronestyl* and *lidocaine* are used less frequently for digitalis-induced arrhythmias.

- The use of the defibrillator for ventricular tachycardia is usually not recommended when digitalis toxicity is present unless the arrhythmia does not respond to drugs or is accompanied by circulatory collapse, because the electrical shock causes potassium to migrate out of the cells and increases the degree of digitalis toxicity. Digitalis effect should not be confused with digitalis toxicity. Digitalis normally causes depression of the ST segments with T wave changes. These effects may be anticipated in most patients who are being digitalized and are not a sign of toxicity.

CARDIAC ARREST

18

The abrupt cessation of effective heart function may be caused by electrical failure with no impulse formation (cardiac asystole or stand still), or ventricular fibrillation with ineffective impulse formation and muscle fiber contraction.

SYMPTOMS

Cardiac arrest is either preceded or quickly followed by cessation of respiration. The signs of cardiopulmonary arrest are:

1 *Pulselessness.* The femoral pulse is usually the most helpful in the determination of the absence of a pulse
2 Cessation of respiration
3 Dilation of pupils within 45 to 60 sec
4 Absence of arterial blood pressure
5 EKG pattern of asystole or ventricular fibrillation
6 Development of body flaccidity

Biological death occurs when the lack of oxygen to the cells with the resultant anaerobic glycolysis has proceeded to the state of irreversible deterioration in the brain and heart [115]. Arterial blood loses 7 percent of its oxygen per minute when it does not circulate. Thus in a patient who previously had a normal oxygen saturation of 96 to 98 percent it takes approximately 4 min for the arterial blood to give up its oxygen and become the same as venous blood. However, if there has been respiratory insufficiency with a decrease of oxygen saturation before the arrest, the length of time after cessation of the circulation of oxygenated blood and biological death is much shorter. Therefore the nurse needs to be skillful both in avoiding the conditions that precipitate a cardiac arrest and in initiating resuscitation measures promptly if cardiac arrest occurs.

Although the responsibility for the treatment rests with the physician, most states have joint statements from the nursing, medical, and hospital associations delegating emergency care to the nurse when the doctor is not immediately available. The medical staff of each individual hospital should also formulate an emergency policy for that hospital. Special training given to the nurse in the interpretation of the EKG and the use of special equipment as a defibrillator or pacemaker should be documented in her file.

CAUSES

Factors that may precipitate a cardiac arrest are:

1 Inadequate circulating blood volume
2 Abnormal levels of electrolytes, especially potassium
3 Vagal stimulation, which may result from prolonged periods of suctioning
4 Valsalva maneuver, which may result when patient holds his breath as he is turned or strains at stool
5 Respiratory insufficiency, since hypoventilation results in an irritable, anoxic myocardium and a predisposition to life-threatening arrhythmias.

VENTRICULAR TACHYCARDIA

The most dangerous arrhythmia is ventricular tachycardia, in which the ventricle takes over the pacing of the heart. Ventricular premature extrasystoles may predispose to the development of ventricular tachycardia, especially when they are frequent, with six or more occurring per minute; are multifocal rather than from the same focus; and they occur during the vulnerable period of repolarization of the ventricles.

Diagnostic Signs

Although ventricular tachycardia is usually preceded by ventricular extrasystoles, it may develop suddenly with no previous ventricular systoles. Sometimes when there have been no preceding PVCs, the EKG pattern of ventricular tachycardia is difficult to differentiate from that of an atrial tachycardia with aberrant conduction. Since digitalis is often given for atrial tachycardia but is contraindicated for ventricular tachycardia, and ventricular tachycardia may progress within a matter of minutes to ventricular fibrillation, it is important for the nurse to know the diagnostic signs of ventricular tachycardia.

EKG

The EKG diagnosis is based on:

1 Heart rate of 130–180/min.
2 QRS widened more than 0.12 sec.
3 P wave and atrial rate independent of ventricular rate and rhythm. (Sometimes an esophageal lead or a pacer electrode in the right atrium will help establish that the P waves have no relationship to the QRS.)
4 Rhythm slightly irregular, with a variation in distance between the R waves of as much as 0.04 sec.
5 Presence of ventricular "capture" beats or fusion beats.
6 Previous EKG showing a PVC which looks like present rhythm.
7 Alternating height of the EKG.

Clinical Features

Clinical features of ventricular tachycardia may include:

1 Hypotension
2 Syncope, especially if there is an impairment in the blood flow to the brain such as occurs with cerebral arterial sclerosis
3 Gastrointestinal ischemia

4   Angina, due to decreased blood flow to the heart

5   Focal neurological signs, caused by inadequate blood flow to the brain

Bedside Diagnosis

The bedside diagnosis may include:

1   The use of carotid sinus pressure, which may affect atrial tachycardia but will not alter ventricular tachycardia since there are no vagal fibers in the ventricles

2   Observation of the neck veins for *(a)* presence of Cannon waves, or *(b)* dissociation of venous pulsations in the neck veins from the apex beat

3   Alternating intensity of the first heart sound

4   Changing height of systolic blood pressure

Treatment

In addition to correcting any underlying cause as respiratory insufficiency or digitalis toxicity, the treatment of multiple ventricular extrasystoles and/or tachycardia usually involves the use of a myocardial depressant drug. A bolus dose of a drug such as lidocaine is usually followed by a slow drip of the drug. Propranolol may be given instead of lidocaine when digitalis toxicity is present. (Drugs and dosages are given in another section.) All antiarrhythmic drugs may cause some type of cardiotoxicity.

If the physician is present, he may elect to terminate a ventricular tachycardia by electric countershock rather than using myocardial depressant drugs [116]. If the patient has shown signs of digitalis toxicity, depolarization is usually not attempted as an elective procedure until a pacemaker can be placed, since the electrical shock causes potassium to migrate out of the cells and increases the degree of digitalis toxicity, which could give a complete block of the AV node resulting in cardiac asystole. Myocardial depressants can also result in asystole if the patient already had a complete heart block. Vasopressors such as Aramine may be given if hypotension is present since the use of Isuprel to raise the blood pressure may increase the irritability of the ventricles and result in another attack of tachycardia.

STEPS IN CARDIOPULMONARY RESUSCITATION

Open-heart surgery patients usually are monitored continuously for their EKG and arterial blood pressure during the early postoperative period, therefore ventricular fibrillation or cardiac standstill can be detected promptly. After cardiopulmonary arrest has been identified, the nurse should waste no time in initiating resuscitation measures. If the patient does not have EKG electrodes and arterial pressure transducers in place, the nurse should identify the arrest on the basis of pulselessness, apnea, and dilated pupils and call for help rather than wasting time in attempting to get an EKG or blood pressure reading. The National Research Council has suggested the use of the following steps in cardiopulmonary resuscitation [117]:

A   Airway

B   Breathing

C   Circulation

D   Diagnosis and definitive therapy
     Diagnosis by EKG
     Defibrillation
     Drugs

This procedure may be deviated from since if ventricular fibrillation is confirmed by the EKG, or is highly suspected, electrical defibrillation may be done immediately if the equipment is available and ready at the bedside. If such is not the case, the usual procedure would be followed.

Airway Restoration

Airway restoration is done by clearing the mouth of any debris or loose dentures and tilting the head backward while pulling up on the jaw. If spontaneous respiration does not resume, an oral airway should be inserted.

Respiration

Respiration is best maintained by the use of a breathing bag such as an Ambu bag, although if a bag is not immediately available, expired air ventilation may be given mouth to mouth. A piece of tubing attached to the Ambu bag and an oxygen outlet will supply a higher concentration of oxygen. Respirations should be assisted at a rate of 12 per minute. Some physicians feel that the rescuer should keep one hand firmly on the abdomen of a patient who is not intubated to prevent air from going into the stomach. As soon as possible, it is advisable to intubate the patient with a cuffed endotracheal tube, since more oxygen is delivered to the lungs and the danger of aspiration from vomitus is lessened.

Circulation

Circulation can sometimes be reestablished by one or two sharp thumps on the chest, if arrest is due to asystole. If heart beat does not return, cardiac compression is indicated. In the absence of a doctor, the nurse will initiate external cardiac compression. However, this method is of limited effectiveness in a patient who had a sternum-splitting incision and whose pericardium had been left open, so equipment should be readied for opening the chest and open-heart massage when the physician arrives. The technique for closed chest compression is included in Appendix C. Indicators that compression is effective are the presence of a palpable femoral pulse and constriction of previously dilated pupils.

In some areas, a machine that takes over both of the functions of assisting respiration and cardiac compression is used. The advantages of a machine are that the rate and force are more constant and it frees the two rescuers for other activities (Fig. 18–1).

When open-chest massage is used, respiration by machine or bagging needs to be continued at the same ratio as used for closed chest compression. There will be no bleeding when the initial incision is made if arrest is present, but bleeding will occur as circulation is restored and will need to be controlled. The nurse can assist the doctor by frequently checking for the presence of a femoral pulse and nondilatation of the pupils.

Defibrillation

Defibrillation for ventricular fibrillation has already been mentioned. The electrical current causes simultaneous depolarization of all the cells in the heart that may allow the normal pacemaker, the sino-atrial node, to regain its dominance and result in restoration of normal rhythm. If the chest has been opened, internal defibrillator paddles may be used by the physician. External defibrillators may employ either direct current (dc) or alternating current (ac). The

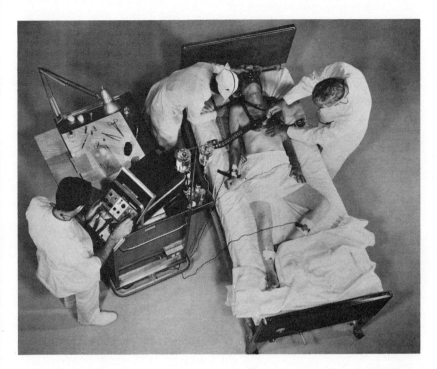

FIGURE 18–1   Heart-lung resuscitator unit in use. This unit can be obtained separately or with the emergency cart pictured. The cart has a swivel-action base to wheel it quickly to the bedside and contains a monopulse defibrillator with an electrocardioscope and pacemaker. The cart also contains a pull-up IV stand, suction machine, high-intensity lamp, bedboard, electrical outlets, and storage for IV solutions and drugs. *(Photograph courtesy of Travenol Laboratories, Morton Grove, Ill.)*

dc defibrillator is generally considered more effective. It delivers a higher voltage over a short period of time. Guidelines for the use of the dc defibrillator are included in Appendix C.

Defibrillation will rarely be successful unless the fibrillation has a rapid rate and a minimum amplitude of 1 microvolt. When the fibrillation is slow with a low amplitude, the myocardium is hypoxic and acidotic, and these conditions must be corrected before defibrillation can be successful. When cardiac asystole rather than ventricular fibrillation is present, defibrillation will not restore the heart beat. Artificial pacemakers may be of value if the asystole is caused by a complete heart block with ventricular standstill or some postoperative condition. If the standstill is due to hypoxia, the heart will not respond to the stimulus of an artificial pacemaker. (The use of a pacemaker is discussed more fully in Chap. 16.)

Drug Therapy

Drug therapy has the following major goals:

1 *To elevate the perfusion pressure. Epinephrine* is usually the preferred drug. One milliliter of 1:1000 solution is usually diluted with 9 ml normal saline to give a 1:10,000 solution. It can be given by IV push directly into the left ventricle, or into the endotracheal tube if the patient is intubated. It has been found to be as effective when given into the endotracheal tube as intravenously [118]. Dosage needs to be repeated every 5 to 10 min. Injections into the heart can result in pneumothorax, myocardial infarction, or puncture of a coronary vessel. *Isoproterenol* (Isuprel) is thought to be more effective than epinephrine by some physicians. Dosage is 0.1–0.2 mg every 3 to 5 min. *Metaraminol, Levarterenol,* and other vasoconstrictor drugs may be used to raise the blood pressure.

2 *To counteract the metabolic acidosis* that results from the lactic acid, pyruvic acid, and other metabolities accumulating in the muscle. *Sodium bicarbonate* given intravenously at a rate to supply 44.6 mEq every 5 to 10 min is usually recommended. (A 50-cc ampoule of 7.5 percent $NaHCO_3$ or 75 cc of a 5 percent sodium bicarbonate solution supplies 44.6 mEq.) Some studies have shown that the progression of acidosis following cardiac arrest is unpredictable, and the amount of bicarbonate required to maintain the pH within normal limits varies. Patients with severe metabolic acidosis accompanied by severe respiratory acidosis were found to profit very little by sodium bicarbonate administration alone, but needed measures to improve ventilation [62]. The drawing of arterial blood immediately after cardiac arrest and the use of a volume-cycled respirator in addition to bicarbonate administration and chest compression for patients who demonstrate marked hypercapnia may become the treatment of choice. Pressure-cycled respirators are ineffective when used with cardiac compression since they are tripped by the compression and recycle without filling the lungs.

3 *To improve the myocardial tone. Calcium chloride,* 5 to 10 ml of a 10 percent solution injected intravenously or into the left ventricle. It is of special value when the arrest is due to a high level of potassium. Calcium gluconate may be given instead of calcium chloride, but the latter is generally preferred because it ionizes faster.

4 *To treat any abnormal heart rhythms* in order to prevent recurrence of fibrillation. The use of myocardial depressants such as Lidocaine and propranolol has already been discussed. If the EKG shows marked slowing of electrical activity, atropine 0.4 mg IV may be given and repeated every 15 min.

POSTRESUSCITATION CARE

This is very important to prevent a recurrence of cardiac arrest. Sometimes respirations and even cardiac compression need to be assisted for a prolonged period of time. When cardiac activity has resumed and the patient is able to maintain his blood pressure over 60 mm Hg, external cardiac compression should be discontinued. The blood-gas values indicate the need for continued oxygen and assisted or controlled ventilation. A chest x-ray may be indicated to determine any injury during the period of cardiac compression and the presence of atelectasis, aspiration, or congestion. Drugs to maintain blood pressure, increase myocardial tone, and control abnormal heart rhythms are continued as needed. Cerebral edema may prevent the patient from returning to consciousness. Sometimes moderate hypothermia and urea intravenously are used to reduce intracranial pressure and control the development of cerebral edema. Dexamethasone may also be effective in reducing cerebral edema.

Discontinuance of resuscitative efforts is indicated if clinical death is irreversible. Jude and Elam [119] cite three signs that indicate there is not sufficient undamaged myocardium to function to keep the patient alive: (1) inability to defibrillate or to maintain defibrillation after repeated shocks, (2) failure of myocardial function or cardiac output after reversal of fibrillation, and (3) lack of improvement in cardiac electrical or mechanical function over a 1-hr period.

19

PROBLEMS

Improvements in heart valve prosthesis, better surgical techniques, and prophlylactic use of anticoagulants (after the chest tubes are removed) to maintain a prothrombin time of 20 percent have decreased the incidence of complications associated with heart valve prosthesis. Some complications that may occur are:

1 Dislodgement of the valve.

2 Rupture of the suture line.

3 Regurgitation, which may be caused by leaks around the sewing ring.

4 Fibrin clots on the prosthesis, which may result in embolic episodes if they become dislodged.

5 Infection, discussed in the section on infections.

6 Ball variance of ball-valve prosthesis. The silastic ball may change in both size and consistency. (Fig. 19–1).

7 Heart block, following suturing of the bundle of His during surgery.

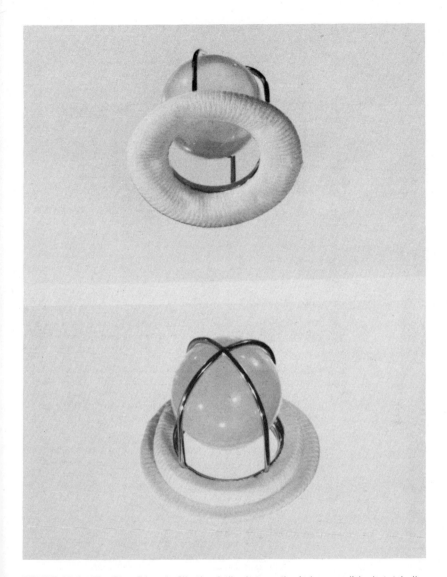

FIGURE 19-1 The Starr-Edwards Silastic™ ball-valve prosthesis has a polished metal alloy cage with a cloth sewing ring. The ball is made of silicone rubber with 2 percent barium for radiopacity. *(Photograph courtesy of Edwards Laboratories, Santa Ana, Calif.)*

8 Trauma to red cells, resulting in hemolysis and chronic anemia. Transient anemia is an expected aftermath of cardiopulmonary bypass. During the first five days after surgery, even with no intrathoracic bleeding, hemoglobin levels may drop as much as

3.5 gm. However, recovery usually occurs by the sixteenth postoperative day [120]. Ten to fifteen percent of the patients have a protracted hemolytic anemia, which is thought to be due to damage to the red cells caused by intracardial or intravascular turbulence that accompanies a leaking valve, especially when the regurgitant lesion is in a prosthetic aortic valve [121].

NURSING ASSESSMENT

Nursing assessment and aids to diagnosis include:

- Close observation of the arterial pressure wave form. After an aortic valve prosthesis, there should be a distinct dicrotic notch which represents the closing of the aortic valve.

- Monitoring of the EKG for signs of heart block.

- Continual assessment for signs of embolic episodes, infection, or heart failure.

- Phonocardiograms done early in the postoperative period as a baseline for follow-up studies. Phonocardiograms can demonstrate: increase in size of ball valve, which is best evidenced by a deterioration or muffling of the opening and closing valve sounds; mitral valve prosthesis murmur; and aortic diastolic murmur.

- Blood studies to detect the presence of traumatic hemolytic anemia. Findings that are considered significant include: low hematocrit, high reticulocyte count, decreased serum haptoglobin, and shortening in red cell survival time (studies made with chromium 51).

TREATMENT

Treatment depends on the problem and its severity. If the size of the ball has increased so the valve fails to operate adequately, or if dislodgement or severe regurgitation occurs, the valve will have to be replaced. Dr. Cooley does not believe that hemolytic anemia alone is an indication for reoperation, since the majority of patients can be maintained on oral iron therapy, with a few patients needing parenteral iron [122]. It is important to avoid functional damage to the renal tubules from the precipitation of hemoglobin resulting from the hemolysis of blood. Fluids are usually forced to maintain a large urinary output to flush out the hemoglobin.

HEART TRANSPLANTATION

20

FOUR MAJOR PROBLEMS

Heart transplants are offering a last desperate hope to persons who are totally incapacitated. Although patients with severe pulmonary hypertension with elevation of pulmonary vascular resistance to systemic levels are not good candidates for heart transplantation, many persons with arteriosclerotic heart disease and cardiomyopathy have an opportunity for increased survival and productivity [123]. In the early stages, four major problems in heart transplantation were identified: (1) surgical technique for transplantation, (2) performance of the heart after denervation, (3) extracorporeal preservation of the graft, and (4) allograft rejection.

The first three problems have been fairly well solved. The surgical method developed by Dr. Shumway does not replace the entire heart in the recipient but leaves the posterior walls of the right and left atria and a thin rim of the posterior atrial septum. Anastomoses of the several veins are combined into one long atriotomy on the right and another on the left, with preservation of both sinoatrial nodes [124] (Fig. 20–1).

It has been found that the cardiac output returns to normal within 2 or 3 days in spite of denervation of the heart. Although

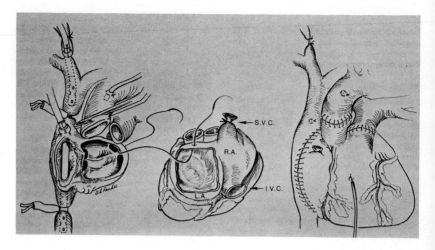

FIGURE 20–1 At left and center, the recipient bed and the donor heart are shown prepared for anastomosis. In the recipient, cannulae are in place in the superior and inferior vena cavae and ascending aorta. Caval tapes and the aortic cross clamp isolate the heart from circulation. The donor heart is prepared by opening out the atria. At right, the anastomosis has been completed and the cannulae removed. A temporary pacing wire is sewed to the anterior right ventricle. *(From R. B. Griepp, E. B. Stinson, D. A. Clark, and N. E. Shumway, A Two-Year Experience with Human Heart Transplantation, California Medicine, 113 (August 1970). Used by permission.)*

there are some slight defects in performance, renervation occurs in 6 to 12 months so the heart eventually responds again to stimuli from the central nervous system.

The problem of extracorporeal preservation of the graft from the time it is removed from the donor until reconstitution of the coronary flow from the recipient was solved by immersing the heparinized donor heart immediately upon excision in saline at 4 to 6°C, which maintains viability of the myocardium up to 6 hr. Following completion of the left atrial anastomosis, the recipient pericardial wall is irrigated continuously with iced saline to provide continued cooling of the dependent portions of the ventricles until coronary circulation is reestablished [125].

The remaining hurdle to be solved is that of homograft rejection. Much of the hope for the future rests on the development of a system of induced tolerance aimed at inducing "immunological paralysis" in the recipient against antigens of the donor. This would result in the recipient not fighting the alien organ, but still having the ability to fight other invaders which could cause disease and infection. Although presently there does not appear to be a correlation between survival and the closeness of the match for histocompatibility, the severity of episodes of rejection has been found to be roughly proportional to the number of tissue antigen mismatches, so the recipient with the closest match is usually selected [123].

INDICATIONS OF EARLY TRANSPLANT REJECTION

Surgeons at Stanford University Hospital have identified three contraindications in the use of a donor heart for a particular recipient [123]:

1 ABO blood group incompatibility
2 A positive cross match between recipient serum and donor lymphocytes
3 Gross difference in the heart size of the donor and recipient

Although there is not total agreement on the reliability of certain signs as indicators of early transplant rejection, those generally accepted by most authorities are:

- Electrocardiogram and vectorcardiogram changes:
  Decrease in the strength of the voltage (amplitude) of the R wave in the limb and precordial leads
  Right axis deviation
  Atrial arrhythmias
  Conduction abnormalities
- Ultrasound signals
  Increased left ventricular posterior wall thickness and stiffness
  Right ventricular dilatation
  Increase in heart size as it fills with fluid
- Hematological findings
  Rise in CBC
  Increase in LDH and other serum enzyme levels
  Increase in lymphocytes
  Rising sedimentation rate
- Pericardial friction rub
- Diastolic gallop rhythm either at the apex or in the left parasternal region
- General malaise
- Easy fatigability

- Rapid pulse with narrowed pulse pressure and paradoxical pattern
- Fever
- Tachycardia
- Oliguria with intractability to diuresis

Chronic rejection, which has resulted in deaths of patients after 6 months, is believed to be evidenced by the progressive narrowing of the coronary arteries by intimal proliferation and fibrosis [123].

MEDICAL AND NURSING MANAGEMENT OF A PATIENT

The usual management of a patient following homograft transplantation includes:

1 The use of drugs to suppress the body's immune mechanism. The drugs include:

(a) *Corticosteroids* for their anti-inflammatory action. Prednisone is given in doses of 60 to 100 mg daily and tapered to 20 to 25 mg daily by time of discharge.

(b) *Azathioprine* (Imuran) is started the day of surgery and continued indefinitely at as high a dose as is compatible with adequate bone marrow function, which is usually 50 to 175 mg a day.

(c) *Antilmphocyte globulin* (ALG). ALG is a serum prepared by injecting a horse with human white blood cells. The horse builds up antibodies against these cells. When the globulin containing the antibodies is given to the recipient of the new heart, the patient's own white blood cells are less effective in fighting his new heart, and the rejection danger is decreased (126). Antithymocyte globulin (ATG) is being tested experimentally at Stanford in place of ALG and it appears to delay the onset of the first rejection episode and allows a reduction in the dosage of other drugs. Usually a maintenance dose of drugs is given, and when the signs of early rejection are detected, the dosage of the drugs is increased until the rejection crisis is over. The first signs of rejection usually do not appear until the sixth or seventh postoperative day. During a rejection crisis, additional drugs are given:

Methyl prednisolone 250–2,800 mg is given intravenously daily.

Actinomycin D (Cosmegen), an antineoplastic drug that also causes hemopoietic depression, is also given daily, 200–750 micrograms intravenously [123].

Systemic treatment with *heparin* is administered during the period of acute rejection because of the higher incidence of intravascular coagulation during rejection [127].

2   In addition to drugs, management of a patient following homo-graft transplantation includes:

•   Use of reverse isolation to reduce the possibility of an infection while the body's resistance is lowered. Gowns, masks, gloves, and surgical boots are worn by all family and personnel for the first 2 or 3 weeks.

•   Emotional support as previously outlined.

•   Teaching the patient and his family good health habits of hand washing, avoidance of injury, wearing clothing that does not rub or chafe, avoidance of scratching or picking of skin, and the like.

•   Careful observation for any signs of infection. Virus infections such as herpes are especially common when the patient is receiving ALG since the cell-mediated response is destroyed.

•   Use of cardiac pacing for 24 to 48 hr while the stroke volume and thus the cardiac output is low to maintain a heart rate of 95 to 110 for the purpose of increasing cardiac output. Atrial pacing is generally the preferred method when there is normal atrio-ventricular conduction [128, 129]. The main advantage of atrial pacing is that the performance of the left ventricle is improved when a properly timed atrial systole precedes the ventricular con-traction, since the atrial systole contributes to ventricular filling. Also, atrial pacing results in fewer extrasystoles. The atrial technique of cardiac pacing is accomplished either by an electrode sutured into the atrial wall medially to the atrial appendage at the time of surgery or by an electrode passed transvenously before surgery and positioned at the junction of the superior vena cava and the right atrium.

•   Use of digitalis and isoproterenol as indicated for their cardiotonic effect.

•   Use of antacids to prevent stress ulcer.

•   Use of Mycostatin as a mouthwash to prevent overgrowth of oral fungi.

- Ambulation on second or third day, with daily physical therapy beginning on the fifth day. A regular regimen of exercise is used to prevent a disabling steroid-induced myopathy. However, activities are limited during a crisis of rejection.

- Observation of other complications of immunosuppressive treatment such as hepatic and bone marrow toxicity, diabetes, osteoporosis, and psychosis.

- Routine for blood, sputum, and skin cultures, blood work (CBC, sedimentation rate, and LDH), exercise electrocardiograms, ballistocardiograms, and ultrasound tracings.

Under laboratory and clinical evaluation is the prophylactic use of an oral anticoagulant and a platelet antagonist such as dipyridamole to reduce the coronary arterial narrowing that has hindered the long-term survival after heart transplantation [123].

POSTINTENSIVE CARE
AND RETURN TO THE COMMUNITY

21

When the critical period is past, and there is no longer a need for the respirator and continuous monitoring, the patient is usually transferred from the intensive care unit. The nurses on the floor to which he goes need to receive a complete report on his condition and any possible problem areas that might require special alertness. The transition is easier if the patient can be returned to the same ward he was on before surgery. If this is not possible, a visit from the nurse who will be his team leader on the new ward helps to ease the natural anxiety he feels over the transfer. The transition is much easier when the patient knows before his surgery that he will be going back to a certain ward, and when the ICU nurse points out his progress and frequently reminds him that at the rate he is progressing, he will soon be well enough that he will not need to be kept in the ICU.

Even with adequate preparation, there is a period of adaptation to the floor care. Many patients need frequent explanation and encouragement to prevent the development of anxiety reactions. The release from the constant surveillance of the ICU is often accompanied by the withdrawal of strong analgesics and tranquilizers, which contributes to the problem of adaptation. As the patient looks ahead to the end of his hospitalized period, problems associated with his home, family, and occupation begin to assume more importance. If the nurse has anticipated these questions and has formed a good interpersonal relationship with the patient, she can help him find realistic solutions to these problems. It is frequently said that planning for effective discharge begins with a patient's admission to the hospital.

The author is engaged in an exploratory study of postoperative heart surgery patients to determine the problems they see as the most difficult in their immediate postoperative period, at three months, and at six months. Many patients are so overwhelmed by the surgical procedure that at the end of two weeks they do not seem to have gathered the emotional resources that will enable them to evaluate their progress and think realistically and constructively about the future. These patients need to rework the surgical experience several times before they are ready to look ahead. If their surgery has not been successful or if complications develop, most patients exhibit symptoms of depression. It appears that those patients who are able to assess their situation realistically two weeks postoperatively place a different evaluation on problems than nursing personnel has historically given. Most patients have felt that pain and dietary limitations are minor problems. Greater problems seem to be in the sociological areas of family relationships. Fear of becoming a burden to the family or of losing one's role and authority are viewed as problems of major importance. Closely related to this is the expectancy of returning to a former job or finding new employment. Patients with pacemakers or prosthetic heart valves appear to require a period of time before they fully accept and trust the operation of their life-sustaining devices.

There has not been adequate time to collect information on the problems that are most crucial to the patients at three and six months after the surgery.

The hospital period should prepare the patient for living at home. Suitable referrals to a public health agency for follow-up care after discharge will ensure that the progress the patient has made in the hospital will be maintained. To prepare the patient to live at home, his postoperative teaching program should include information on activity allowed, medications, diet, and any special restrictions. The amount of responsibility assumed by the nurse for this teaching depends on the physician and the type of hospital setting. If the physician prefers to give certain information himself, the nurse needs to report the patient's questions in this area to the doctor.

NURSING MANAGEMENT

The usual management of patients includes:

Activity

Patients are encouraged gradually to increase their activity, but to postpone moderate or heavy physical activity until a later date when they have been checked out by the physician. Sitting for longer than 2 hours without a little ambulation is discouraged. A rough criterion of ability to resume sexual activity without adverse effects is toleration of a walk of three blocks at a moderate pace.

Medications

Anticoagulants

Patients who have a prosthetic heart valve need to be aware of the importance of the careful and consistent taking of their coumarin drug and of keeping laboratory and/or doctor's appointments for determination of prothrombin time and adjustment of dosage. Prothrombin time is usually maintained at 20 percent. In addition, patients need to know the importance of:

1 Wearing a *Medic Alert* emblem with suitable engraving on the back or carrying a card in their wallet that gives information about their valve and anticoagulant therapy. The engraved emblem has an advantage over the wallet card since it is always with the patient (Fig. 21–1).
2 Avoiding aspirin, steroids, and other anti-inflammatory drugs that interfere with the aggregation of the platelets, and thus with blood clotting.
3 Watching the stools, gums, and so on for any signs of bleeding.
4 Reporting to any other physician or dentist about the medication he is taking.

Diuretics

Diuretics may be given if needed to prevent fluid retention. Most physicians prefer not to keep patients on a daily dose unless they have cardiac decompensation or renal damage that makes daily medication necessary. Patients are usually taught to weigh themselves on the

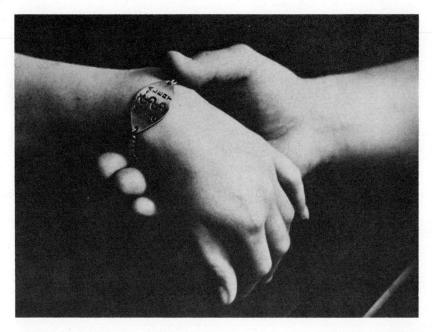

FIGURE 21–1   Medic Alert bracelet for emergency identification. *(Photograph courtesy of Medic Alert Foundation, Turlock, Calif.)*

same scale at the same time every morning and diuretics are only given for an increase in weight of 2 or 3 lb over a 24-hr period.

Digitalis Preparations

These may be given as indicated to improve myocardial competence. A patient on a digitalis drug should know the signs of toxicity that should be reported to the physician before the drug is continued. A period of self-medication under the nurse's supervision before the patient goes home is an effective method of determining his ability to follow directions for medications.

Diet

Diet is often low sodium, low cholesterol. Calories may be restricted for the overweight patient. Patients with athersclerotic heart disease have more rigid restrictions on their diets than other patients. Written instructions (such as a printed list of foods that must be omitted and those that are restricted) should be given as well as verbal instruction.

Some of the guidelines given by the Inter-Society Commission for Heart Disease Resources include [130]:

Products to Use	Products to Avoid*
Lean cuts of meat, poultry, and fish	Fat cuts of meat and processed meat high in saturated fat
Low fat and fat-modified dairy products†	High saturated fat, dairy products, and nondairy cream that contain coconut oil or hydrogenated vegetable oil
Oils and margarine low in saturated fat	Butter, margarine, and shortening high in saturated fat
Grains, fruits, vegetables, and legumes	Egg yolk, bacon, lard, and suet (claims of health food stores that the cholesterol in eggs fertilized by roosters is better assimilated by the body have not been supported by research)

*Patients accept their diet resrtictions more willingly when the reason for the restriction is explained.
†Fat modified refers to products made with reduced saturated fat and cholesterol content.

Special Restrictions

Pacemaker patients need to be alerted to the hazard of entering an area containing microwave generating equipment, e.g., a microwave oven. They also need to be taught to inspect the skin area over the module and take their pulse daily. A slowing of the rate below the rate set for the pacemaker may mean battery failure or another problem and the physician should be consulted.

For patients who live in more remote areas, the Cardiac Datacorp, Inc., has a pacemaker evaluation system that diagnoses pacemaker problems from a telephone recording and reports any problem to the physician (Fig. 21–2).

The patient has been found to be less fearful after he has mastered the operation of the pacemaker. The use of role rehearsal of emergency situations and letting him practice dealing with them will increase his self-confidence and feeling of adequacy [131].

EMPLOYMENT BARRIERS

With the increasing trend in many states to include heart conditions under Workmen's Compensation coverage because the condition is said to have been aggravated by overwork, stress of the job, and other emotional factors, employers have been hesitant to rehire an employee with a heart problem [132]. The American Heart Association

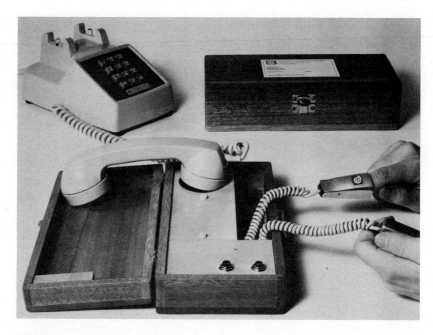

FIGURE 21–2   Pacemaker transmitter in operation. The electrode with the magnet is held in the left hand, and the right index finger is placed in the sensing electrode. The telephone mouthpiece is placed over the hole in the panel for transmittal. The operator may ask the patient to put the magnet over the pacemaker module if the pacemaker is suppressed by the patient's QRS. (Magnet makes the pacemaker operate as a fixed-rate pacer.) *(Photograph courtesy of Cardiac Datacorp, Inc., Philadelphia.)*

has an ad hoc Committee on Stress, Strain, and Heart Disease that is working to improve this situation. Some suggestions made by the Committee at the 44th Scientific Sessions were that the second injury law should be expanded to include cardiac cases, that state legislatures should decide what claims are compensable, and that testimony of cause of illness should be given by a cardiologist or internist. Another suggestion is that disability or some other type of insurance be instituted to cover the hazards of simple aging and chronic disease [132].

CONTINUITY OF CARE

It has been estimated that 25 percent of the adults who undergo heart surgery will need a follow-up by the Public Health Nurse when they return to the community [133]. These patients may require both physical and psychological rehabilitation. The local chapter of the

American Heart Association can usually supply information on resources and types of assistance available locally for the cardiac patient. Many hospitals have social service workers who are available for counseling and making arrangements for and with patients. However, it is important for the nurse also to know of the various programs so she can answer questions posed by the patient or his family and reinforce the information given by the social worker. Programs available in most areas are: Program of Vocational Rehabilitation under the State Board of Education; information on employment and job training from the State Department of Employment and many local agencies; services of a visiting nurse, home health aide, or Public Health Nurse; work evaluation unit of the American Heart Association or other sponsor that offers testing of the patient's functional capacity; and local chapter of The Mended Heart, Inc., which is founded to help and encourage persons who need or have had heart surgery.

When the patient is dismissed from the hospital, the nurse has the responsibility of recording the patient's condition at discharge, state of all incisions, activity tolerance, and any teaching or referrals that were made.

APPENDIX

A

Table of Major Heart Defects and Their Surgical Correction

Name	Description	Diagnostic Aids	Surgical Procedure
Aortic valve defects:		*All aortic valve defects* Left ventricular enlargement EKG findings of left ventricular strain Angina caused by decrease in coronary blood flow X-ray may show calcification of aortic valve Syncope and heart failure	
(1) Aortic stenosis	Obstruction to blood flow through aortic valve caused by fusion and decreased flexibility of leaflets of aortic valve. May be congenital or acquired as a result of rheumatic valvulitis, syphilis, or subacute bacterial endocarditis.	Loud, harsh systolic ejection murmur in 2d intercostal space with transmission into neck and a palpable thrill over neck and chest. Pressure gradient across aortic valve of approximately 100 (left ventricle higher than aorta). Sound of aortic valve closure decreased or absent. Notched brachial artery pressure curve with a prolonged rise time.	For congenital or when there is no aortic calcification, with use of bypass, median sternotomy and horizontal aortotomy are performed. Commissures are incised almost to the annulus. Valve replacement indicated for severe stenosis and calcification; Starr-Edwards ball-valve prosthesis usually used.

(2) Idiopathic hypertrophic subaortic stenosis	Congenital condition caused by fibrous ring below aortic valve in outflow tract that contracts during systole and almost occludes outflow tract.	Symptoms similar to aortic stenosis with cineangiographic views that may show subaortic hypertrophy.	Excision of hypertrophied fibrous tissue through a ventriculotomy incision while on cardiopulmonary bypass.
(3) Aortic insufficiency	Incompetent closure of aortic valve resulting from deformity of aortic valve leaflets and/or dilatation of aortic annulus. Deformity caused by the same factors as in stenosis. Dilatation of annulus may be caused by aneurysms of ascending aorta and cystic medial necrosis (with or without Marfan's syndrome).	Blowing murmur in early diastole in 2d intercostal space and along left sternal border. Wide pulse pressure of water-hammer type (distension followed by rapid collapse). Fluoroscopy shows a widely pulsating aorta. Cineangiographic injection of contrast media into aorta shows appearance of media in ventricles.	Valve replacement while on temporary cardiopulmonary bypass.
Atrial septal defect	Congenital, functionally significant opening between right and left atrium. Most common type is incompetent foramen ovale. Other defects may occur high in the septum (persistent ostium secundum) or low in the septum (persistent ostium primum). Low septal defects may be associated with mitral or tricuspid valve defects. Ten to fifteen percent of patients also have anomalous pulmonary connections. Since pressure is normally higher in left atrium than in right atrium, flow of blood is usually from left to right except when severe cases result in pulmonary vascular hypertension.	Soft systolic murmur at pulmonic area and diastolic murmur at tricuspid area. x-ray shows small aorta, blooded lungs, right ventricular enlargement, and small left atrium. EKG findings of axis deviation, incomplete right bundle branch block, and left and right ventricular hypertrophy. Acyanosis, except in severe cases of lung damage and pulmonary hypertension in which shunt is from right to left. Cardiac catheterization shows an increase in oxygen saturation in right atrium over superior vena cava.	Atriotomy under bypass through median sternotomy incision with closure of defect by direct suture of patch graft from pericardium. Valve defects or anomalous veins must be corrected if present.
Coarctation of aorta	Congenitally occurring narrowing or constriction of lumen of aorta, which occurs as either preductal or postductal obstruction, depending on position in relation to ductus arteriosus (Fig. A-1).	Upper extremities may be better developed than lower extremities. Coldness and pulselessness of lower extremities. Hypertension, with systolic BP much lower in legs than in arms.	Through a left lateral thoracotomy incision, aorta is dissected free, clamped proximally and distally, and narrowed segment resected, with anastomosis of proximal and distal segments. Graft may be required if

Table of Major Heart Defects and Their Surgical Correction *(Continued)*

Name	Description	Diagnostic Aids	Surgical Procedure
		Aortogram shows aortic indentation. Barium swallow may show esophagus displacement. X-ray shows notching of ribs caused by enlarged collateral vessels.	resected section is long. In small children, room for growth is provided by interrupted sutures. Advantageous to perform operation on older children because segment used as graft will not grow as aorta does.

POSTDUCTAL COARCTATION

COARCTATION OF THE AORTA

FIGURE A–1

Coronary artery
disease

Disease of coronary arteries that may be
generalized narrowing caused by atherosclerosis or narrowing of a segment
only, with resultant myocardial
ischemia in area affected.

Coronary arteriography, with injection of
contrast medium into each of the three
coronary arteries to visualize arteries
and extent of collateral circulation.

Revascularization (modified Vineberg
procedure) using unilateral or bilateral
mammary artery implants into tunnels
in myocardium for diffuse coronary
artery disease.

Treatment of choice is aortocoronary
bypass procedure utilizing grafts from
saphenous vein for narrowed or
occluded segments of coronary
arteries (Fig. A-2). Within short
period of time, patency of grafts has
been found to be 82 percent [134].
Patients with severe generalized distal
coronary artery occlusive disease are
not good candidates for surgery.

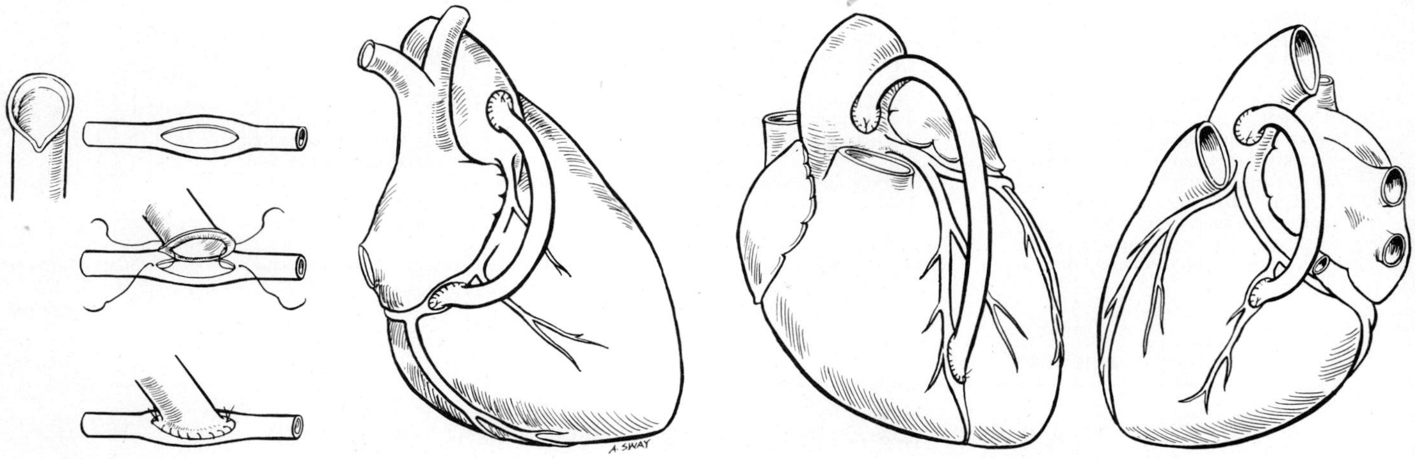

FIGURE A-2 Artist's conception of end-to-side anastomosis of vein grafts to coronary artery. Common sites of right and left anterior descending and lateral marginal branch of the circumflex coronary vein graft anastomosis. (*Reprinted by permission from the New York State Journal of Medicine, copyrighted by the Medical Society of the State of New York, Surgical Treatment of Coronary Artery Insufficiency, vol. 71, no. 14, July 15, 1971, and by permission of the author, Robert G. Carlson, M.D., Department of Surgery, New York Hospital.*)

Table of Major Heart Defects and Their Surgical Correction (Continued)

Name	Description	Diagnostic Aids	Surgical Procedure
Mitral valve defects:			
(1) Mitral stenosis	Narrowing of mitral orifice, resulting in increased resistance to blood flow from left atrium to left ventricle. Sometimes congenital, but usually results from rheumatic inflammation that leaves the cusps of valves thickened and commissures fused.	Left atrial hypertrophy. Right ventricular enlargement as decompensation progresses. Diastolic murmur at apex with opening snap following closely on 2d heart sound. EKG findings of strain, left atrial hypertrophy, and often atrial fibrillation. Hemoptysis, systemic emboli, atrial thrombi. Cardiac catheterization shows increased left atrial pressure and normal left ventricular pressure with pressure gradient across mitral valve. Pulmonary artery pressure is elevated, and there may be pulmonary congestion and edema. Cineangiography shows stiff, funnel-shaped valve on diastole.	Midline sternotomy done, and if feasible, valve repaired. Mitral valvulotomy can be done with closed-heart procedure by finger dilation, valvulotome, or transventricular dilator, but these methods are rarely used. Plastic repair usually done under direct vision with bypass. When atrial thrombus, mitral regurgitation, or much calcification is present on valves, valve prosthesis is usually indicated. Although all artificial valves have imperfections, Starr-Edwards ball-valve prosthesis usually used. Disk valves, with very little exposed metal, that will decrease thrombosis on prosthesis and peripheral embolization are being tested experimentally.
(2) Mitral insufficiency	Impairment of closure of mitral valve, with leakage or regurgitation, which usually accompanies mitral stenosis. May also be caused by rupture of chordae tendineae, rupture of papillary muscle secondary to myocardial infarction, or dilated valve annulus caused by previous episodes of left ventricular failure.	Left atrial and left ventricular hypertrophy. EKG shows left ventricular hypertrophy, sometimes PVCs. Harsh systolic murmur at 4th or 5th intercostal space. Cardiac catheterization shows increased left atrial and left ventricular pressure. Cineangiographic injection of contrast medium into left ventricle shows simultaneous appearance of medium in left atrium and aorta.	Ruptured chordae tendineae can be repaired by suturing involved portion of valve to papillary muscle. Valve may need to be replaced.

Myocardial aneurysm	Outpouching of myocardial wall, especially of left ventricle, that occurs following myocardial infarction. In Ebstein's malformation there is aneurysmal dilation of right ventricle, with atrial septal defect creating atrialized right ventricle from aneurysm.	Fluoroscopic examination may demonstrate paradoxical motion of myocardium during systole since functioning portion of ventricle contracts while aneurysm fills with blood and dilates. May have systemic embolization from mural thrombus in aneurysm. Cardiac catheterization shows enlargement of ventricle involved.	Through thoracotomy incision, with use of cardiopulmonary bypass, aneurysmal pouch is excised with margin of fibrous tissue left to hold sutures placed to close ventricular defect. In Ebstein's malformation, tricuspid valve usually needs to be replaced also.
Patent ductus arteriosus	Vascular connection that normally closes shortly after birth, which, if it fails to close, shunts blood continuously from aorta into pulmonary artery (Fig. A–3).	Continuous machinery murmur heard high on the chest wall under left clavicle. Cardiac thrill in 2d interspace that may radiate.	Surgical division of ductus through left thoracotomy incision with closure of two ends, which closes openings into pulmonary arteries and aorta. Can be done without cardiopulmonary bypass

PATENT DUCTUS

FIGURE A–3

233

Table of Major Heart Defects and Their Surgical Correction (*Continued*)

Name	Description	Diagnostic Aids	Surgical Procedure
		Acyanotic unless pulmonary artery pressure exceeds 130, in which case shunt is reversed. Increased pulse pressure. Angiography visualizes the patent ductus.	bypass. Usually done when child is between 3–8 years old.
Pulmonic valvular stenosis	Congenitally narrow pulmonary valve, usually accompanied by poststenotic dilatation of pulmonary artery and may be associated with septal defects. Infundibular stenosis is diffuse muscular hypertrophy of outflow tract of right ventricle that constricts the tract but usually found only in conjunction with other abnormalities.	Loud systolic murmur and thrill at 2d intercostal space with diminished or absent pulmonic sound. Cardiac catheterization shows higher systolic pressure in right ventricle than in pulmonary artery, and angiography will show dilation of pulmonary artery. EKG shows right axis deviation and right ventricular hypertrophy. X-ray films show decrease in pulmonary circulation. Cineangiographic studies outline pulmonary valve bulging into pulmonary artery on systole.	Any hypertrophied muscle present is cut away. Valve is opened by incising it along line of fused commissures.
Tetralogy of Fallot	Congenital anomaly that presents four defects: ventricular septal defect; aorta overriding (straddling) septal defect, thus receiving blood from both ventricles; pulmonic stenosis; and right ventricular hypertrophy (Fig. A–4).	Cyanosis. Faint systolic murmur present almost from birth. Body size small and health poor. Clubbing of fingers at an early age. Squatting after exertion. Episodes of paroxysmal dyspnea and syncope. X-ray of heart shows bootlike appearance with bulge of left heart border and undercirculated lung fields.	Palliative shunt procedure to divert blood from aorta into pulmonary artery for infants too small for bypass (modified Blalock). Correction includes median sternotomy and, while on bypass, incision in right ventricle through which pulmonary stenosis is corrected and ventricular defect repaired. Pulmonary valve may need to be replaced.

TETRALOGY OF FALLOT

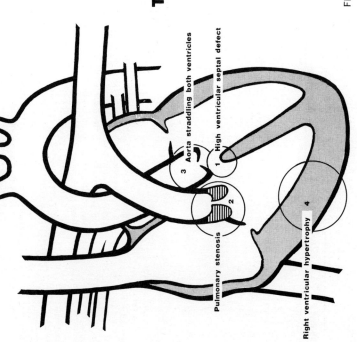

3 Aorta straddling both ventricles

1 High ventricular septal defect

Pulmonary stenosis 2

Right ventricular hypertrophy 4

FIGURE A-4

235

Table of Major Heart Defects and Their Surgical Correction (*Continued*)

Name	Description	Diagnostic Aids	Surgical Procedure
Transposition of the great vessels	Congenital defect in which aorta originates from right ventricle and pulmonary artery from left ventricle (Fig. A–5).	EKG shows right axis deviation and right ventricular hypertrophy. Blood count may show polycythemia. Cyanosis. Rapid increase of heart size, with egg-shaped contour. X-ray of lung shows normal or increased vascularity. May have systolic murmur. Clubbing and polycythemia. Cardiac catheterization shows increased oxygen saturation in right heart and oxygen saturation in pulmonary artery higher than systemic saturation.	Most surgical procedures are palliative operations to increase crossflow of blood between arterial and venous circulations, such as creation of atrial septal defect. Some procedures have attempted to transpose completely inflow of blood into left atrium so left and right sides of heart are reversed in their activity.
Tricuspid valvular disease: (1) Tricuspid stenosis	Uncommon condition, usually resulting from rheumatic fever, in which valve leaflets are fused and chordae and papillary muscles are deformed. Usually occurs with mitral and aortic valve disease.	EKG shows hypertrophy of right atrium, frequently atrial fibrillation. Cardiac catheterization shows higher pressure in right atrium than in right ventricle. Signs of systemic venous engorgement. A diastolic murmur in 4th interspace increased with inspiration. Giant A wave in the jugular pulse.	With cardiopulmonary bypass, valvuloplasty or valve replacement.
(2) Tricuspid insufficiency	Leakage around the tricuspid valve caused by deformity of valve leaflets or by dilatation of annulus of valve, which may result from dilatation of right ventricle with right-sided heart failure.	Cineangiography shows regurgitation in right atrium of contrast medium from right ventricle. Systolic murmur in 4th or 5th interspace that increases with inspiration. EKG shows right atrial hypertrophy, right axis deviation, right ventricular hypertrophy.	Tricuspid regurgitation may disappear if right ventricular function is improved. With bypass procedures, severe cases may be treated by valvuloplasty, annuloplasty, or valve prosthesis.

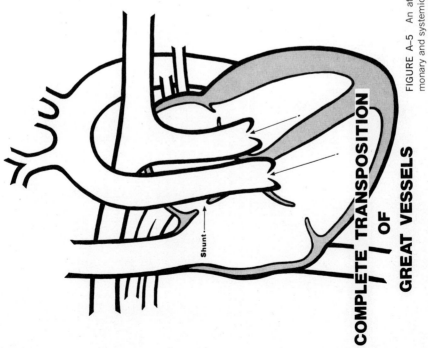

COMPLETE TRANSPOSITION

OF

GREAT VESSELS

Shunt

FIGURE A–5   An atrial septal defect or other abnormal communication between the pulmonary and systemic circulation must be present to sustain life.

Table of Major Heart Defects and Their Surgical Correction *(Continued)*

Name	Description	Diagnostic Aids	Surgical Procedure
(3) Tricuspid atresia	Congenital absence of opening between right atrium and right ventricle for flow of blood, which requires presence of atrial septal defect for survival. Often associated with pulmonary stenosis, which further limits oxygenation of blood.	Cyanosis. Underdeveloped right ventricle. Cardiomegaly. Undercirculation of pulmonary vasculature.	No procedure for correction, but artificial shunt to provide more pulmonary blood flow is helpful.
(4) Ebstein's malformation	Congenital defect involving the tricuspid valve, an atrial septal defect, and frequently aneurysm of the right ventricle.	Cyanosis. Dilatation of the right atrium. Cardiac angiograph shows deformed and displaced tricuspid valve and flow from right atrium into left atrium. EKG shows axis deviation and frequently Wolff-Parkinson-White syndrome.	While on cardiopulmonary bypass, repair or replacement of valve, closure of atrial septal defect, and plication of aneurysm.
Truncus arteriosus	Congenital condition in which aorta receives blood from both ventricles, the blood from right ventricle passing through high ventricular septal defect.	Cyanosis of varying intensity. Variable murmurs: continous murmur usually present. Enlarged heart.	No effective operation at present.
Ventricular septal defect	A congenital abnormal opening in septum between right and left ventricle. Since pressure is usually higher in the left ventricle, blood passes from left to right side of the heart during contraction. If pulmonary hypertension and high pulmonary vascular resistance are present, blood will be shunted mainly from right to left ventricle, resulting in some unoxygenated blood passing into general circulation.	Loud systolic murmur noted as early as 2 weeks of age. X-ray picture of enlargement of right ventricle and large pulmonary artery, with increased vascularity of lung fields.	Small asymptomatic defect does not require closure. For child too small for bypass, temporary procedure in which a band is placed around the pulmonary artery is sometimes done. Permanent repair is through median sternotomy or transverse incision; on cardiac bypass, defect is sutured or repaired with Teflon patch graft. (Pericardium not used for graft because of possibility of aneurysm from high vascular pressure.)

238

| Ventricular septal defect (Eisenmenger's) syndrome | Eisenmenger's syndrome—essentially large ventricular septal defect with severe pulmonary hypertension resulting in a major shunt from right to left. | Cyanosis may be present when shunt is from right to left. | When shunt is from right to left with irreversible changes in pulmonary vascular bed and pulmonary hypertension, surgery not generally recommended since with defect closed there is no outlet into systemic circuit for high right ventricular pressure, and pulmonary edema will result. |

APPENDIX

B

Chart of Most Commonly Used Cardiovascular Drugs

Drug	Characteristics	Therapeutic Use	Usual Dosage	Contraindications or Signs of Toxicity
		Cardiotonic		
Isoproterenol (Isuprel)	Inotropic Chronotropic Beta adrenergic Peripheral vasodilator Increases conduction in AV node Bronchodilator	Cardiogenic shock Advanced stages of heart block Bradycardia For quinidine toxicity Bronchospasm	1 to 2 mg in 500 cc IV fluid given with a microdrip 0.1 to 0.2 mg as bolus dose or into left ventricle every 3 to 5 min 0.5 ml of 1:200 solution in nebulizer	Ventricular extrasystoles Tachycardia Should not be administered simultaneously with vaso-constrictive drug such as epinephrine because heart is then forced to "beat against a brick wall"
Epinephrine (Adrenalin)	Inotropic Alpha and beta adrenergic Increases coronary blood flow Decreases peripheral resistance (in most patients)	Cardiac arrest	1 mg IV bolus. 0.5 to 1 mg given into left ventricle [dilute 1 ml of 1:1000 (1 mg) with 9 cc of saline to give 1:10,000 dilution, and give 5 to 10 cc]	Tachycardia Ventricular extrasystoles
Digitalis	Inotropic Slows conduction time in AV node	To increase cardiac output For control of such supra-ventricular arrhythmias as	Intravenous preparation Des-lanoside (Cedilanid D) 1 to 2 mg initially with 0.2 mg	Caution should be used when giving to any patient with AV block

Drug	Action	Indications	Dosage	Comments
	Depresses SA node Increases refractory period in atria and ventricle	flutter, fibrillation, and tachycardia	every 1 to 2 hr Ouabain 0.1 to 0.5 mg. Very quick acting, but action lasts only 30–45 min Oral or intramuscular Digoxin (Lanoxin) 2 to 4 mg for digitalization, 0.5 mg for maintenance Digitoxin 1 to 2 mg for digitalization, 0.1 mg for maintenance	Toxic signs include: heart block, tachycardia, nodal rhythms, bigeminal rhythm, PAT with block, anorexia and nausea, visual disturbances, headache, lethargy
Atropine	Vagolytic since depresses parasympathetic nervous system Shortens refractory period of AV node	Sinus bradycardia, especially with rates below 50 For incomplete AV block	0.4 to 1.2 mg by IV bolus; may be repeated every 1 to 4 hr	Should not be given to patients with glaucoma May cause urinary retention
Calcium chloride	Increases cardiac muscle tone	Cardiac arrest, if arrest is caused by high potassium level or by a myocardial depressant such as lidocaine	0.5 to 1 gm IV (5 to 10 ml of 10 percent solution) into left ventricle or as IV bolus. May be repeated every 8 to 10 min if necessary	Should not be given to patients with digitalis toxicity, since it increases toxic effect Should not be added to solutions containing sodium bicarbonate since calcium carbonate may be formed
Adrenocorticosteroids	Inotropic alpha adrenergic blocker Increases filling pressure of the heart	Cardiogenic shock Septic shock	Intravenous preparations—hydrocortisone (Solu-Cortef) 250 to 3000 mg Methylprednisolone (Solu-Medrol) 125 to 1000 mg repeated as often as every 2 hr Dexamethasone (Decadron) 4 to 100 mg every 8 hr IV If given for less than 3 days may be discontinued abruptly. Longer periods of	A preexisting ulcer may start to bleed. Diabetes may be aggravated since steroids speed conversion of glycogen to glucose in the liver

Chart of Most Commonly Used Cardiovascular Drugs (Continued)

Drug	Characteristics	Therapeutic Use	Usual Dosage	Contraindications or Signs of Toxicity
		Cardiotonic		
			therapy require gradual reduction of dosage	
Glucagon	Inotropic Chronotropic Decrease in vascular resistance Increase in AV conduction	Cardiogenic shock (equivocal)	5 to 10 mg IV push every 15 minutes; 15 mg IV over 1 hr	Diaphoresis Hypokalemia Nausea
3, 4-Dihydroxy-phenylethy-lamine (Dopamine)	Inotropic Chronotropic Alpha adrenergic action on blood vessels of skeletal muscles Nonadrenergic renal and mesenteric vasodilatation	Cardiogenic shock (experimental use of drug)	0.5 to 10 micrograms per kg per minute IV [135]	Unknown at this time
		Myocardial Depressants*		
Lidocaine (Xylocaine)	Myocardial depressant Decreases myocardial contractile force	Ventricular tachycardia Ventricular extrasystoles	25 to 100 mg IV bolus followed by continuous drip with 4 gm in 1000 cc to eliminate more than 5 extrasystoles/min (or original dosage can be repeated after 10 min if necessary)	Seizures Respiratory arrest (Ritalin 10 mg given to counteract unless on automatic respirator) Conduction defects may be an adverse reaction
Procainamide (Pronestyl)	Procaine derivative decreases myocardial irritability	Ventricular tachycardia and extrasystoles	0.3 to 1 gm IV bolus given at rate of 100 mg per min,	Hypotension, particularly on standing

Drug	Action	Use	Dosage	Toxicity
	Slows sinus rate Depresses AV conduction and intraventricular conduction	Atrial tachycardia	followed by IV continuous drip that gives 5 to 10 mg per min (1000 mg in 500 cc IV) 250 to 500 mg by mouth every 6 hr for maintenance	Widening of QRS more than 50 percent is indication for stopping drug
Propranolol hydrochloride (Inderal)	Beta adrenergic blocker Prolongs refractory period of AV node Blocks bronchodilator effects of catecholamines	Supraventricular tachycardia Ventricular extrasystoles Ventricular tachycardia Used when digitalis is contraindicated because of digitalis intoxication	1 to 5 mg IV at rate not to exceed 1 mg/min. Oral administration preferred, 10 to 30 mg 4 times a day	Bradycardia Bronchospasm Hypotension Decreases contractility of heart and blocks catecholamine-stimulating effect, so not given if congestive heart failure is present, or to postoperative patients unless digitalis toxicity is present
Quinidine	Vagolytic Slows conduction time in the AV node Depresses SA node Decreases myocardial irritability and contractility Vasodilator	To decrease conduction in AV node To decrease ectopic contractions in both atria and ventricle and reduce possibility of chemically induced fibrillation To convert atrial fibrillation, but should give digitalis first to block AV node so the increase in impulses through AV node will not result in ventricular fibrillation	IV drug rarely given. May give 300 to 500 mg over a period of 30 to 60 min Orally 1 to 4 gm in divided doses over 24 hr Maintenance dose 0.8 gm daily in divided doses	Hypotension Thrombocytopenia Headache Nausea, vomiting, diarrhea Tinnitus, visual disturbance, and deafness Lengthening of QRS complex more than 25 percent Mural thrombi may be dislodged from atria when atrial fibrillation reverts to normal rhythm
Diphenylhydantoin (Dilantin)	Decreases ventricular automaticity May improve conduction through the AV node (equivocal)	To counteract ventricular tachycardia caused by digitalis toxicity, sinus tachycardia when digitalis is contraindicated	250 mg diluted to 25 mg/ml given IV over 5–10 min Maintenance 200 to 600 mg in divided doses (IM or by mouth) over 24-hr period	Hypotension Bradycardia

Chart of Most Commonly Used Cardiovascular Drugs (Continued)

Drug	Characteristics	Therapeutic Use	Usual Dosage	Contraindications or Signs of Toxicity
Myocardial Depressants*				
Edrophonium chloride (Tensilon)	Vagotonic	Prevention of ventricular fibrillation when hypothermic Conversion of paroxysmal atrial tachycardia	10 mg by IV bolus	Bradycardia
Bretylium tosylate (experimental drug)	Decreases ventricular irritability Positive inotropic action	Ventricular tachycardia Ventricular extrasystoles. May be successful in converting ventricular fibrillation that is resistant to multiple countershocks [136] PAT	300 to 600 mg IM or IV 300 mg every 6 to 8 hr for maintenance	Depletes catecholamines Postural hypotension Diarrhea Nausea and vomiting (nausea worse with IV administration)
Vasoconstrictor (vasopressor) Drugs†				
Metaraminol (Aramine)	Predominantly alpha adrenergic Peripheral vasoconstrictor	To raise BP in shock due to hypovolemia	5 to 10 mg IV bolus; 50 to 250 mg added to 500 cc IV fluid and run at a drip to maintain desired BP	May cause sinus bradycardia If used over a period of several days will deplete body's catecholamines, so unable to wean from drug. Switching to Levophed for 24 hr will let body build up store of catecholamines
Levarterenol or norepinephrine	Predominantly alpha adrenergic with intense	As a last resort to maintain BP	16 to 32 mg (8 to 16 ml) added to 500 cc 5 per cent	May cause sinus bradycardia If infiltration occurs, Regitine

244

(Levophed)	peripheral vasoconstrictive action Coronary vasodilator		D/W to run at a slow drip to maintain desired BP Regitine may be added to IV infusion	should be given sub-cutaneously in areas of infiltration to prevent tissue slough

Vasodilator Drugs

Chlorpromazine (Thorazine)	Alpha adrenergic blocking agent	To decrease peripheral vaso-constriction Antiemetic Tranquilizer	4 to 16 mg IV every hour as needed	Jaundice (rare)
Phentolamine (Regitine)	Alpha adrenergic blocking agent	To reduce peripheral vasoconstriction Increase tissue perfusion Decrease pulmonary congestion	5 mg IV. Duration of action is short, so usually 75 mg added to IV fluid given over 24 hr	Tachycardia, hypotension due to rapid expansion of vascular space Rapid administration may impair myocardial contractility
Phenoxybenza-mine (Dibenzyline)	Alpha adrenergic blocking agent	Same as phentolamine	1 mg/kg given slowly over a 1-hr period	Same as phentolamine

*If the EKG shows AV dissociation, no myocardial depressant should be given until pacemaker is installed or cardiac arrest may result.
†All peripheral vasoconstrictor drugs used over a period of time dispose to metabolic acidosis.

APPENDIX

C

Guidelines for Nursing Procedures

Steps in Procedure	Rationale
	Blood Gas Analysis

Heparinize a glass 10-ml syringe by drawing up 1 to 2 ml heparin (1000 units per ml) and slowly pulling plunger back to 10-ml mark on barrel. Then, while holding syringe with needle pointing upward, slowly push plunger all the way in, ejecting any excess heparin.	Unclotted blood is needed for the blood gas analyzer.
Withdraw 10 ml blood from arterial line, using plain syringe. Then withdraw 10 ml into heparinized syringe, being careful to avoid bubbles. If arterial line is not in place, specimen must be obtained by arterial puncture.	First blood withdrawn from catheter is diluted with IV fluid, so another sample is withdrawn for analysis (Fig. C–1).
Immediately expel any air from the arterial sample by holding syringe upward and squeezing plunger until air is expelled.	Air mixed with blood distorts true gas content.
Stick needle into a cork and rotate syringe gently.	Cork prevents air from entering syringe, and rotation prevents clotting.
If unit does not have a blood gas analyzer, place syringe in container of crushed ice and send it promptly to laboratory.	Use of ice retards blood cell metabolism.
Record information concerning use of a respirator and flow of oxygen with blood gas report.	Information is necessary for accurate evaluation of blood gas data.

Guidelines for Nursing Procedures *(Continued)*

Steps in Procedure	Rationale
	Measurement of Central Venous Pressure (CVP) with a Water Manometer
Prepare bottle of IV fluid and attach central pressure tubing	Tubing should be purged of air and ready to connect to patient as soon as venous catheter is placed, to prevent clotting of blood in catheter.

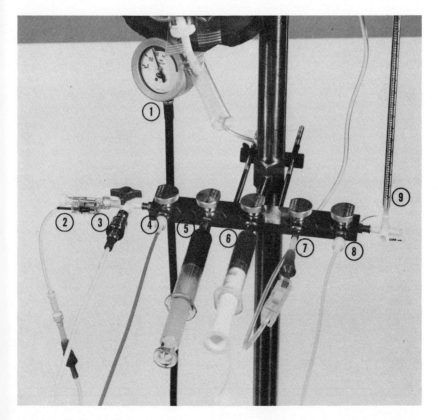

FIGURE C–1   Polymanifold setup for monitoring and blood gas analysis. Plastic syringe (No. 6) is used to withdraw fluid and blood mixture from arterial line. Glass syringe (No. 5) is used for pure blood sample. Other items in photograph include (1) pressure infusor around plastic bag of heparinized fluid. Pressure on bag is maintained above 200 mm Hg to maintain arterial drip. (2) "Intraflow," a commercially available continuous flush system. By pulling on the black rubber stem, rapid flushing of the arterial line is facilitated without adjustment of the slow maintenance drip rate. (3) Arterial transducer. (4) Arterial line. (7) CVP fluid line. (8) Central venous line. (9) CVP manometer. Note that stopcocks on the CVP side are set for infusion (with the CVP manometer off) and on the arterial side the transducer and flush line are turned off with the arterial catheter open to the glass syringe during specimen withdrawal.

Guidelines for Nursing Procedures *(Continued)*

Steps in Procedure	Rationale

Measurement of Central Venous Pressure (CVP) with a Water Manometer

including water mano- meter and three-way stopcock. Mount manometer on IV pole, and with stopcock turned to cut off mano- meter, fill tubing with fluid, making sure all air is removed. Attach tubing to CVP infusor or intracath into patient's vein. Open clamp to allow fluid to drip slowly.	
Label site CVP and tape to secure position. Use arm board or tongue blade (for jugular vein puncture) if indicated.	Bending of tubing with flexion of the arm or movement of the head must be prevented.
Place patient in recumbent position and mark level of right atrium on his chest with a felt-tip pen. Right atrium is located inferior to midsternum and one-half distance between anterior and posterior chest walls.	To get accurate right atrial pressure reading, reference position for right atrium must be established.
Place zero (0) level of manometer at level of patient's right atrium by using leveling instru- ment or removing manometer from IV pole and holding it against chest.	For accuracy, each reading must be taken with same reference position.
Allow a few ml of fluid to run in rapidly and then turn three-way stopcock to cut off line to patient and observe fluid as it rises in manometer. Do not allow fluid to over- flow manometer.	Flushing tubing before taking reading helps maintain patency and accuracy. Since top of manometer is open to air, it can become contaminated. Fluid should be kept a few cm below top of tube to reduce chance of infection.
Turn three-way stopcock to cut off line from intra- venous bottle. Observe column in manometer; should fall rather quickly until it reaches stable	Hydrostatic pressure in manometer equalizes with patient's venous pressure. Inaccurate readings are commonly caused by obstruction to lines or kinks in system (e.g., lateral flexion of neck toward site of needle in external jugular vein or flexion of arm at needle site in antecubital fossa can obstruct flow of fluid).

Guidelines for Nursing Procedures *(Continued)*

Steps in Procedure	Rationale

Measurement of Central Venous Pressure
(CVP) with a Water Manometer

point. Level in mano-
meter should fluctuate
slightly with each
respiration.

Take reading at eye level,
using maximum of
meniscus after level
becomes stable (Fig.
C–2). Notify physician
of any malfunction.

Obstruction can be detected by slowness in reaching equilibrium and
by absence of effect of respiration on pressure. If level fluctuates
widely with heart beat and reading is high, catheter may have
slipped into right ventricle where it can cause abnormal heart
rhythms.

Turn stopcock to shut off
manometer and allow
solution to run from IV
bottle to patient.
Regulate flow as
ordered.

Fluid must drip slowly into system at all times except when reading is
being taken to prevent line from becoming clotted with blood.

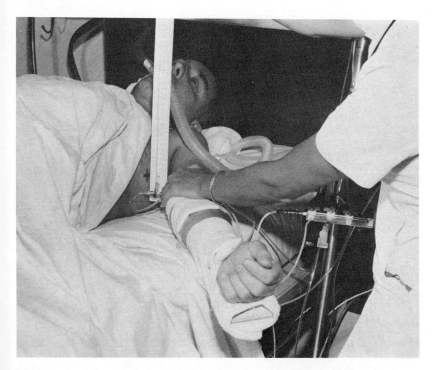

FIGURE C–2   One method of measuring the central venous pressure, with the zero on the
manometer placed at the level of the right atrium.

Guidelines for Nursing Procedures *(Continued)*

Steps in Procedure	Rationale

Administration of Closed Chest Compression

Place board approximately 30 by 30 by 1 in. under patient's chest.	Rigid surface is needed to secure adequate compression.
Position yourself at patient's side at height that allows your hands to rest on his chest with your arms straight.	Proper height is necessary for administration of adequate pressure.
Place heel of one hand on lower third of sternum just above xiphoid process and parallel with long axis of patient's body. Place second hand on top of first.	Proper placement of hands is important to prevent unnecessary rib fractures or trauma to liver.
Exert downward pressure on sternum until it is depressed 1½ to 2 in. toward spine, depending on size of patient. Thrust should be delivered rapidly and then released.	Adequate pressure squeezes heart between sternum and backbone, pushing blood into circulation. When pressure is released, chest wall recoils and heart can fill with blood.
Continue compression at rate of 60 times a minute. Pause between every fifth compression for assisted respiration. If only one person is available for both cardiac compression and ventilation, use ratio of 12 compressions to 2 respirations.	Circulation of blood without adequate provision for oxygenation will be ineffective.
Evaluate effectiveness of resuscitation by ascertaining presence of femoral and peripheral pulses and constriction of previously dilated pupils.	Evaluation of effectiveness is essential to determine whether resuscitation efforts should be continued.

Use of the Defibrillator

With machine turned "off," plug it into electrical outlet and then activate "on" switch.	When machine is on, it is ready to accept current; therefore spark may occur as terminal prongs are plugged into electrical outlet.

Guidelines for Nursing Procedures *(Continued)*

Steps in Procedure	Rationale

Use of the Defibrillator

If defibrillator has synchro-nizer, turn synchronizer off for patient in ven-tricular fibrillation.	Leaving synchronizer on would cause defibrillator to wait to dis-charge at peak of R wave, and there is no R wave in ventricular fibrillation.
Set dial for watt-seconds of electricity desired. Many physicians prefer to start with low-energy level around 200 watt-seconds.	Use of lowest energy level that will result in depolarization for patient prevents unnecessary burns and other cellular damage.
Apply conductive jelly to both paddles, being careful that jelly does not extend over edge of paddles. Alternate method: Place saline pads on chest where electrode paddles will be placed.	Conductive jelly or saline is necessary for conduction of electrical impulse through chest wall and heart.
Place electrode paddles firmly on chest, rotating them a little when con-ductive jelly is being used. Paddles can be placed in various positions as needed, but usual placement for patient without implanted pacemaker is one paddle at apex of heart and other just to right of sternum below clavicle (Fig. C–3).	Rotation of paddles helps to assure good contact. Electricity will flow from discharging electrode paddle to receiving electrode paddle, so paddles must be spaced so current can pass through heart.
Patient with implanted pacemaker should have paddles placed per-pendicular to wires.	Some implanted pacemakers can be damaged by electrical discharge traveling along pacing wires. Damage is minimal when paddles are placed perpendicular to wires.
Turn off EKG machine and disconnect any temporary transvenous pacer that may be in use.	Equipment may be damaged if not inactivated.
Charge defibrillator by pushing button marked "charge." Watch gauge to determine when storage capacitor is fully charged and unit is ready for use.	The charge button activates circuit that charges storage capacitor to preselected energy level.

Guidelines for Nursing Procedures *(Continued)*

Steps in Procedure	Rationale

Use of the Defibrillator

Instruct all personnel to step away from bed and metal equipment.	Anyone touching patient or bed is in danger of receiving shock intended for patient.
Apply 10 to 20 lb firm pressure to paddles and deliver electrical discharge by pushing button on electrode paddle or instructing assistant to depress "discharge" button on machine.	Firm pressure is necessary to assure that electrical current travels through chest wall and heart instead of arcing from one electrode to another.
Palpate femoral artery and restart EKG machine.	Presence of femoral pulse and normal electrocardiographic pattern is evidence of successful defibrillation.

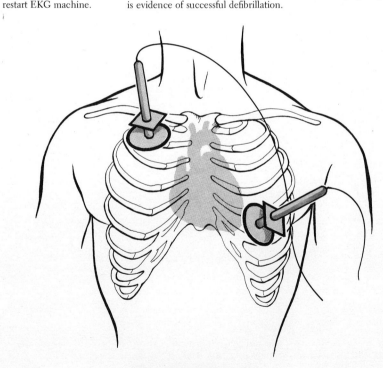

Placement of

DEFIBRILLATOR PADDLES

FIGURE C–3

Guidelines for Nursing Procedures *(Continued)*

Steps in Procedure	Rationale

Use of the Defibrillator

Increase energy level and recharge defibrillator if another attempt at defibrillation is indicated.	Increased energy level may be necessary to effect depolarization. Machine must be recharged after each use.

Suctioning an Endotracheal Tube

With cuff of endotracheal tube inflated, suction oropharynx with large-bore catheter if secretions are present.	Releasing cuff before suctioning oropharynx allows any mucus above cuff to drain into lungs.
With patient still on respirator, deflate cuff gradually. Suction mouth and oropharynx as indicated.	Airway pressure with patient on respirator will force any remaining secretions up into the mouth where they can be suctioned out.
Disconnect patient from respirator, but leave respirator on.	Respirator should be ready for immediate use if patient shows signs of hypoxia.
Slowly instill 2 to 5 ml normal saline into endotracheal tube with a syringe. Keep needle used for withdrawal of saline taped to bottle.	Saline helps to loosen secretions so that they can be suctioned out. Needle should never be used on the syringe because of danger of its dropping off into tube and lodging in lung.
Pour approximately 150 ml sterile saline into clean paper cup.	The author has not found sterile containers for saline necessary or feasible.
Wear a rubber or vinyl glove on the hand that touches catheter. Lubricate a sterile, soft rubber, or plastic whistle-tip catheter by dipping it into saline.	Lubrication with saline and use of soft rubber catheter reduces damage to mucosa.
With the patient's head turned to right and left shoulder elevated, carefully pass catheter down endotracheal tube.	Passage of catheter into left main bronchus is facilitated when patient's head is turned to right.
Attach catheter to suction tubing and apply suction by occluding opening of Y with forefinger or thumb while gently rotating catheter (Fig. C–4).	Catheter can be connected to suction tubing before it is passed, but there is some suction even when Y is open. Thus it is less traumatizing to mucosa to connect catheter after it has been passed.

Guidelines for Nursing Procedures (Continued)

Steps in Procedure	Rationale
	Suctioning an Endotracheal Tube

Do not continue suctioning more than 15 sec at a time. Rotate catheter as it is withdrawn, using intermittent suction.	Prolonged suctioning can remove all available oxygen from bronchus. Suction applied continuously as catheter is withdrawn may pull mucous membrane into catheter with a resultant lesion.
Flush catheter with saline in cup.	Maintains patency of the catheter. Some have recommended changing to a fresh sterile catheter and regloving, but most practitioners have not found this necessary.
If patient shows no signs of hypoxia, reinsert catheter with patient's head turned to left and right shoulder elevated.	To pass catheter into right main bronchus.
Suction in same manner as previously outlined. If patient shows signs of intolerance, place him back on respirator (with 100 percent oxygen when indicated) for a period before further suctioning is attempted.	Some patients develop abnormal heart rhythms that may result in cardiac arrest while being suctioned. Dr. Shim recommends that any patient with tendency to abnormal heart rhythms should receive 100 percent oxygen for 5 min prior to suctioning [137].

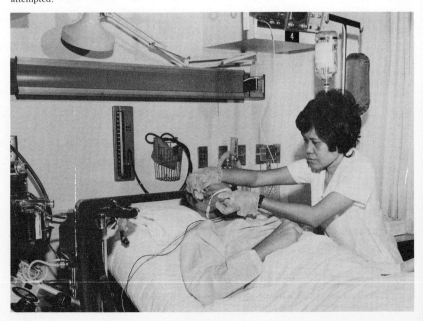

FIGURE C–4 Suctioning an endotracheal tube. The left bronchus is suctioned with the patient's head turned to the right and the opening of the Y occluded.

Guidelines for Nursing Procedures *(Continued)*

Steps in Procedure	Rationale

Suctioning an Endotracheal Tube

If suctioning fails to remove tenacious secretions, occlude opening of tube with sterile gauze square and encourage patient to cough.	Coughing may help raise secretions so they may be reached by the suction catheter. However, because intubated patient cannot close his glottis, he can rarely cough effectively.
When airway is free of secretions, carefully reinflate cuff. Do not inflate it more than is necessary to prevent air from leaking around it.	Overinflation predisposes to pressure necrosis.
Try to get patient to breathe with respirator, and then reconnect him to respirator. Observe for synchronization of respirations with machine.	The author has found that resynchronization with respirator is facilitated when patient is encouraged to match his rate with that of machine.
Discard glove and paper cup. Discard catheter or place it in receptacle for reprocessing.	Use of fresh equipment each time reduces infection.

D

Guidelines for Electrical Safety

Measures	Rationale
Keep electrically susceptible patient isolated as much as possible from any metal surface or equipment that is plugged into electrical outlet.	Patient who has monitor leads with conducting jelly on his chest is susceptible to macroshock (electric current applied to body surface) because his normal skin resistance is lowered. Voltages in excess of 50 may cause ventricular fibrillation in this susceptible patient. Even smaller voltages are hazardous for patient with external pacemaker connected to pacing catheter in heart or a fluid-filled catheter (CVP line) in heart, since these lines provide path for conduction of electricity to heart muscle itself. This current, termed *microshock*, applied internally, may result in ventricular fibrillation if amount exceeds 10 milliamperes.
Do not touch patient while you are in contact with metal surface of an item that is plugged into electrical outlet.	Another person can provide a path of transmission of electric current from equipment to patient without feeling any shock himself.
Discourage use of electric beds until nonmetallic electric beds are available at a reasonable price. If electric beds are used, check them frequently (while bed is being run) for leakage current.	Metallic electric beds have been termed by some engineers the "reclining version of the electric chair." There is normal leakage current in any electrical equipment between hot wire and ground. This leakage is created by capacitance from their proximity and sometimes contributed to by a resistive path caused by poor insulation. If bed becomes ungrounded, this leakage current may flow through patient when he touches bed rail, and could be hazardous for an electrically susceptible patient. To assure that leakage current is held to low level, bed should be tested while motor is running with ac microamperemeter. Leakage current in excess of 100 microamperes is generally considered unacceptable.
Report any unusual electrical interference on EKG recording that cannot be corrected by electrode adjustment. Discontinue use of equipment if interference is limited to one machine.	Interference may indicate possible microshock danger.
If electric shock or tingle is felt when touching item of electric equipment, immediately touch equipment a second time. If shock or tingle is felt second time, disconnect equipment and report to department responsible for electrical engineering safety.	Touching equipment a second time distinguishes between electrostatic discharge and shock hazard, since tingle from electrostatic discharge will not be felt second time.

Guidelines for Electrical Safety *(Continued)*

Measures	Rationale
If electrostatic discharges are experienced, always touch bedframe with a metallic object (e.g., key) before touching patient.	Danger of electrostatic shock is not known, but by touching bedframe with metal object, both patient and nursing personnel are protected from discharge.
Before using any piece of electrical equipment, inspect cord and plug. Do not use equipment with frayed or damaged cord or with plug that is bent or has ground prong missing. *Never* use ungrounded or "cheater" plugs.	When ground wire is not intact, normal leakage current will not flow safely back to power system ground, and leakage current may find another path to earth, which may be through patient who grounds himself by touching oxygen outlet or who is indirectly grounded by nurse who touches him at same time she adjusts his oxygen flow.
Do not use molded plugs. Have any molded plugs on equipment converted to removable-type plugs with ground wire slightly longer than other two wires.	On testing molded plugs, 40 percent of them were found to have defective placement of ground prong [138]. When ground wire is longer than other wires, stresses are taken by hot and neutral wires, and they will fail before the ground wire fails. (Failure of hot or neutral wire will result in nonfunction of equipment while failure of ground wire will not affect function.)
Do not allow any patient-owned electrical equipment (e.g., electric shaver or radio) to be used. Battery-operated equipment may be permitted.	Patient-owned equipment does not usually have grounding system and may have significantly high leakage current.
Do not use extension cords except in extreme emergencies.	For every foot of cable used, leakage current increases. Also, plugging into an outlet not in patient's unit may be risking the danger of difference in ground potential.
Cover any exposed electrodes or uninsulated pacemaker leads connected to patient with rubber or other insulating material.	Contact of electrode or lead with another person or any source of ground or leakage current may cause microshock.
Always wear rubber gloves when connecting or disconnecting externally worn pacemaker.	Connectors of pacing catheter provide conductive pathway to heart and thus make it susceptible to microshock.
Use only equipotential grounding systems (termed *equal potential bus)*, and plug all equipment used for one patient into outlets at his bedside.	When outlets and all metal surfaces in room are tied together to ground terminal, everything around patient has same ground potential, and problem of fault current creating potential difference between two grounds that could result in shock is minimized.
Conduct routine checks on electrical outlets to ensure that plugs fit tightly, wiring ground is intact, and internal connections have not deteriorated.	Commercial testers are available to assess integrity of outlets, which is critical to electrical safety since current may flow through the patient, as previously described.

Guidelines for Electrical Safety *(Continued)*

Measures	Rationale
Use monitoring equipment that has current-limiting capability. Current should not exceed 10 microamperes. Older equipment that does not limit current should be modified or used with isolation unit (Fig. D–1).	Isolation units are designed to protect patient from any current above 10 microamperes that may occur between him and monitor, without interfering with operation of monitor.

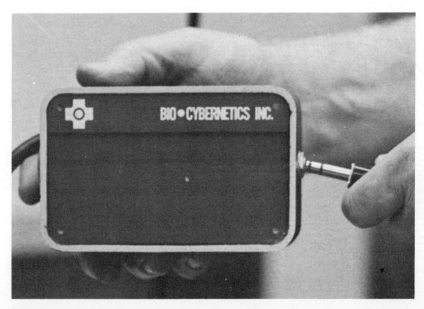

FIGURE D–1 ISOLATION UNIT. The cable from the patient electrodes is being plugged into the isolation unit. The other cable is plugged into the monitor. This unit is designed to protect the patient from any current above 10 μA that may occur between the patient and the monitor. *(Photograph courtesy of Bio Cybernetics, Inc., Watertown, Mass.)*

Note: Credit for much of the above material is given to F. J. Weibell and E. A. Pfeiffir [138].

E

Electrocardiographic Tracings with Interpretations

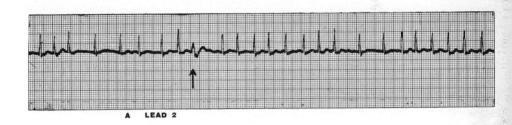

A LEAD 2

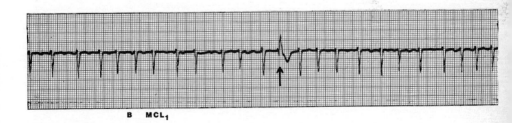

B MCL₁

FIGURE E-1   Atrial fibrillation with a rapid, irregular ventricular response and occasional aberrant ventricular conduction. It is important to distinguish aberrance from premature ventricular beats (PVB's) because the administration of lidocaine, procaineamide, or quinidine may facilitate conduction in the AV node and increase the heart rate. The major factors that delineate aberration are: (1) Triphasic *RSR'* pattern in *MCL₁*. (Eighty percent of all aberrant beats resemble right bundle branch block.) (2) The initial deflection in right bundle branch aberrant conduction is always positive in *MCL₁*. (3) It occurs primarily when a long cycle is followed by a short cycle. The long cycle lengthens the following refractory period, and with the right bundle branch still refractory, it is conducted aberrantly, resembling a right bundle branch block.

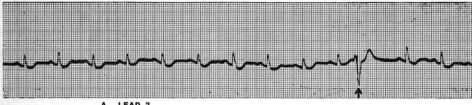

A LEAD 2

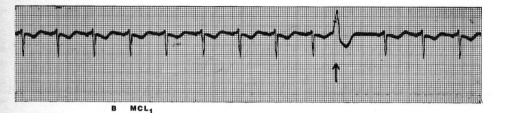

B MCL₁

FIGURE E–2   Sinus rhythm of 75/min with premature ventricular beats (PVB's). Since the ectopic beat in *MCL*₁ has a *qR* pattern, it probably originated in the left ventricle. (Right PVB's have a *rS* configuration.) The following characteristics of a PVB are present: (1) Occurs early; (2) is not preceded by a p wave; (3) is widened of bizarre configuration and shows altered repolarization; (4) is followed by a compensatory pause.

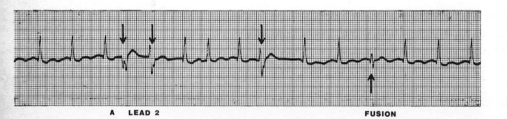

A LEAD 2   FUSION

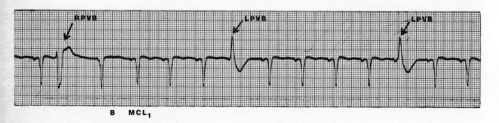

B MCL₁

FIGURE E–3   Sinus rhythm of 75/min with multifocal PVB's in a patient following a ventricular aneurysectomy. *MCL*₁ indicates that PVB's are from both right (*rS* configuration) and left (*qR* configuration) ventricle. One fusion beat is present on Lead II. Lidocaine was given for such frequent PVB's.

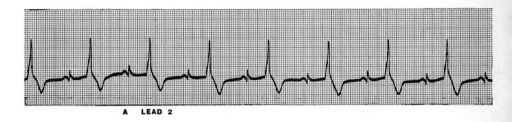

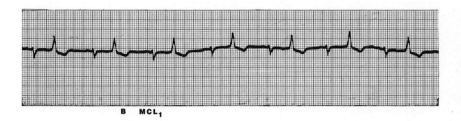

FIGURE E–4   Ventricular bigeminy in a patient with intraventricular block. Since the beats conducted from the sinus node are widened and the R wave is very small in *MCL₁*, this block may be of the left bundle branch variety. *MCL₆* validated this speculation. Every other beat is a ventricular premature beat that is coupled to the preceding sinus beat. In this patient, the cause of the bigeminy was digitalis toxicity.

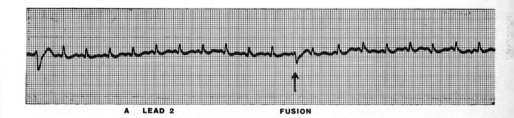

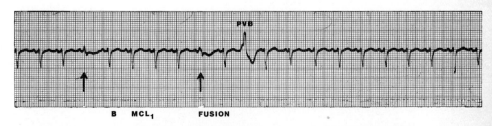

FIGURE E–5   Sinus tachycardia with a rate of 120/min with PVB's and fusion beats. The fusion beat results when a sinus beat partly depolarizes the ventricles at the same time an ectopic ventricular focus is depolarizing another part of the ventricles, giving a complex midway between a normal supraventricular beat and a ventricular beat. In most cases this establishes the ventricular origin of the latter part of the beat.

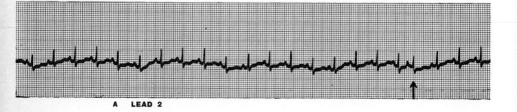

A   LEAD 2

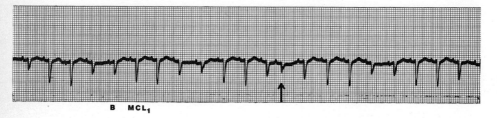

B   MCL₁

FIGURE E–6   Sinus tachycardia of 125/min with occasional premature atrial beats (PAC's). The premature beats are determined to be supraventricular based on the criteria that the ventricular depolarization *(QRS)* is not changed and the pause is not fully compensatory. The change in height of the *QRS* complex is caused by the movement of the chest with respiration.

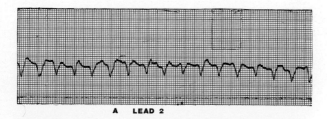

A   LEAD 2

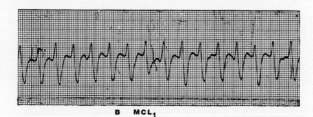

B   MCL₁

FIGURE E–7   Ventricular tachycardia of 150/min. Factors aiding the diagnosis are p waves that bear no relationship to the *QRS, QRS* complex 0.14 sec wide, and the rate of 150. The clinical picture of hypotension and syncope contributed to the diagnosis.

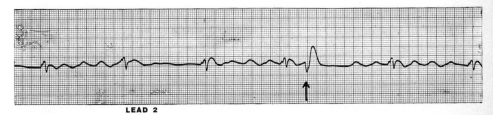

LEAD 2

FIGURE E-8 Idioventricular rhythm with a rate of 34/min in a patient in cardiogenic shock. The *QRS* complex is widened and bizarre. The variation in the baseline is artifactual. The beat indicated by the arrow is a ventricular ectopic of different origin.

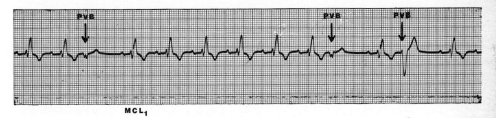

MCL₁

FIGURE E-9 Patient following an aortic valve prosthesis placement with a sinus rhythm and a rate of 80/min. The *pr* interval of 0.24 sec indicates first-degree AV block. There is a triphasic *RSR'* pattern in *MCL₁* with a conduction time of 0.16 sec indicating right bundle branch block (RBBB). Multifocal PVB's are present.

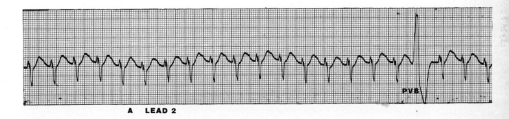

A   LEAD 2

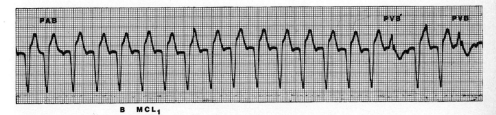

B   MCL₁

FIGURE E-10 Supraventricular tachycardia of 120/min with bundle branch block. Presence of PVB's with a fully compensatory pause and one premature supraventricular beat allows the p wave to be more clearly seen. The block is in the left bundle branch since the *QRS* is 0.14 sec wide and there is no r wave in *MCL₁* (validated by *MCL₆*, which showed a late intrinsicoid deflection without a Q wave).

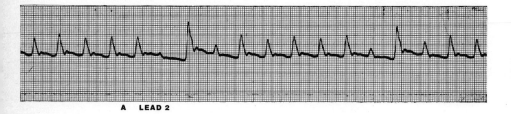

A   LEAD 2

B   MCL₁

FIGURE E–11   First-degree AV block (*pr* interval 0.24 sec). The altered configuration of the *QRS* complexes in Lead II (all of which arrive on time) is artifactural. *MCL₁* has a PVB. There are two possibilities for the wide appearance of the *QRS* in Lead II: one is that the S-T segment is incorporated into it, and the other is that because of the difference in time in recording the two leads, the conduction pattern was altered.

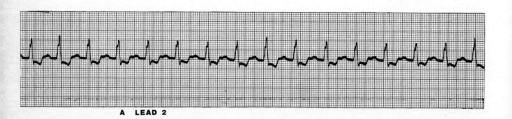

A   LEAD 2

B   MCL₁

FIGURE E–12   Patient 24 hr postaortic valve prosthesis placement. Sinus rhythm of 85/min with first-degree AV block (*pr* interval 0.28 sec) and left bundle branch block (ventricular complex is 0.14 sec and *MCL₁* has no R wave.)

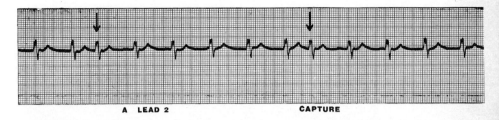

A LEAD 2   CAPTURE

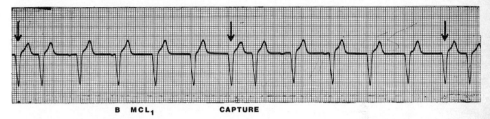

B MCL₁   CAPTURE

FIGURE E–13   Same patient as Fig. E–12, 36 hr postaortic valve prosthesis placement. Patient has now developed complete AV dissociation with a junctional rhythm conducting in the same LBBB pattern. Lead II looks different from the previous tracing because of slightly different electrode placement. P waves can be identified and reveal an atrial rate of 65/min. A junctional (nodal) rhythm of 75/min is seen with capture occurring every sixth beat. (A capture beat is a conducted beat following a period of AV dissociation.)

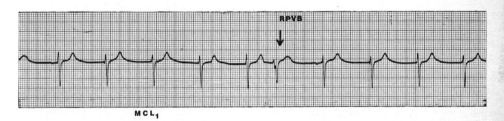

MCL₁

FIGURE E–14   AV dissociation with a slow junctional escape rhythm of 58/min. Atrial rate of 50/min. One premature ventricular beat from the right ventricle is present. The beat following the PVB is probably a conducted beat. The patient should be given atropine if increasing the rate is indicated.

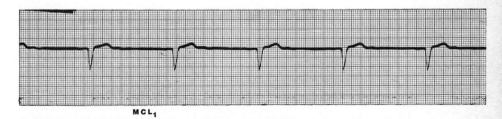

MCL₁

FIGURE E–15   2:1 second-degree heart block with a ventricular rate of 33/min. Atrial rate of 66/min. Every other sinus impulse is blocked, and those conducted have a prolonged conduction time of 0.28 sec. Ventricular depolarization is also prolonged (0.16 sec).

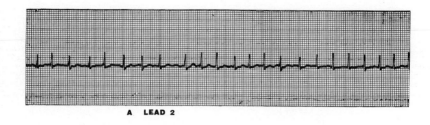

A LEAD 2

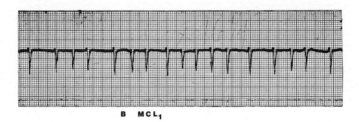

B MCL₁

FIGURE E–16 Atrial fibrillation with a rapid ventricular response in a patient following mitral valve prosthesis. Patient was given intravenous Cedilanid, which successfully decreased the ventricular response.

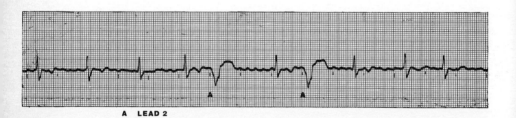

A LEAD 2

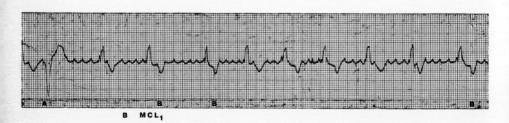

B MCL₁

FIGURE E–17 Atrial flutter fibrillation in a patient with a prosthetic mitral valve and temporary pacing wires sewn on the left ventricle. Wires are connected to a demand pacemaker set at 90/min, but pacemaker is malfunctioning and rarely captures. (The A on the tracings indicates capture by the pacemaker). It can be seen that the pacemaker is not suppressed by the patient's own QRS and occasionally fires near the vulnerable period of the T wave (B on the MCL₁ tracing). Pacemaker should be turned off and the patient observed closely until the problem can be corrected.

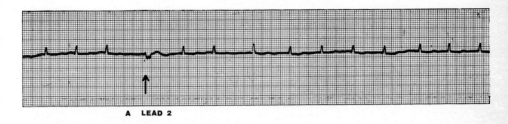

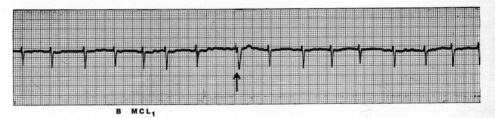

FIGURE E–18 Demand pacemaker in a patient with atrial fibrillation. Pacemaker rate is 75/min, and pacemaker fires and captures the ventricle when no supraventricular impulse is transmitted. (Arrows point to pacemaker capture beats.)

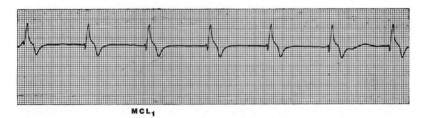

FIGURE E–19 Slow idioventricular rhythm of 45/min. This is a passive ventricular rhythm arising in the left ventricle to rescue the heart that suffers from atrial standstill.

APPENDIX

Sample Nursing Care Plan

Synopsis of history: John Smith is a 49-year-old white male who has had severe angina for the past 6 months. Had stroke 2 years ago with a residual weakness on right side.

Surgery performed: Aortocoronary bypass graft to the right and left anterior descending coronary artery using a saphenous vein graft with extracorporeal circulation.

Patient Need	Approach
Maintenance of adequate ventilation	On Engstrom respirator 6 liters O_2 − 4 liters air Rate = 16 Head elevated 30° Record expired minute volume qh Sigh by ↑ air 2l × 2 resp. qh Instill 2 to 5 cc of NS and suction prn Observe for synchronization with respirator—morphine prn (see ticket) Blood gases q4h 2–6–10
Prevention of pressure necrosis or injury from ET tube	Support respirator tubing Release ET cuff qh Reinflate cuff carefully—approx. 7 cc—avoid overinflation Oral care qh
Conservation of oxygen used for metabolism	Monitor temperature qh Aspirin supp. 0.6 gm for temp ↑ 101°R Cooling blanket for temp ↑ 102°R
Recognition of early signs of inadequate circulation	Continuous monitoring of central arterial pressure. Maintain slow heparinized drip for arterial line. Apical and radial pulse qh Check tissue perfusion (peripheral pulses) qh (R dorsalis pedis not palpable) CVP and LAP qh Level of consciousness qh (R hand grip weak from previous stroke)
Recognition of abnormal heart rhythms	Continuous monitoring of EKG Lidocaine drip (with Ivac) for PVCs ↑ 5/min
Maintenance of fluid volume and electrolytes within normal limits	Foley to Cystoflow drainage. Record urine output, sp. g., and pH qh Save 24 hours urine for K (until 2 pm) Maintain microdrip on IV infusion (1000 cc for 24 hr = 40 cc/hr or 40 gtt/min) Weigh 8 am daily—bed scales
Prevention of venous stasis	Encourage alternate flexion and extension of ankles and flattening of knee to bed Turn q2h—even hours. Have patient exhale as he is turned Antiembolic stocking. Reapply 6 am–2–10 pm

Sample Nursing Care Plan *(Continued)*

Patient Need	Approach
Maintenance of chest drainage for lung expansion	Chest tubes to waterseal drainage. Emerson pump at 20 cm pressure Milk tubes qh Record chest drainage qh—maintain cumulative balance Observe tubing for fluctuation
Prevention of infection	Inspect wound and all arterial and venous puncture sites frequently. Clean and redress infusion sites with neosporin cream prn and daily—10 am Antibiotic q6h via buretrol (see ticket)
Reduction of stress	Wants to be called "John" Give patient his glasses (contain hearing aid) when he is awake Wife can only visit in morning Enjoys having FM transistor radio on 1490 Writes with left hand since his stroke Maintain comfort and rest with morphine and Atarax (see ticket)

APPENDIX

G

Sample of Composite Nurses' Notes for Opean-Heart Surgery Patients

Time PM / AM	BP	P	R	Temp. (R)	Atrial Pressure RAP (CVP)	LAP	Periph. Circ. (Pulses)	IV Intake	Blood Chest Drain	Re-placed	Blood Balance	Urine Amount	Urine sp.g.	pH	Vent. Exp. Min. Vol.	Nurses' Notes
2:10	150/104	84	16	96	14	17	3 +	3000 cc 1750 cc	Blood IV fluid			388				From O.R.
2:30	154/100	84	16	97	14	17	3 +								10	6 Oxygen Engstrom 4 Air
2:45	140/94	86	16													
3:00	138/90	84	16	97.8	13	17	3 +	200 molar lactate	50		−50	100	1.016	6	10	PO_2 148 ph 7.44 PCO_2 42 O_2 sat 98.8
3:15	132/94	90	16				2 +									Blood started
3:30	126/90	88	16	98.2	13	16	2 +		100	200	+50					

Time	BP	Pulse	Resp	Temp			Edema	IV	100 molar lactate		±		Sp. Gr.			Orders / Notes
4:00	110/90	84	16		12	16	2 +					55	1.025	5.5	10.5	MS 3 mg Not synchronized with Engstrom
5:00	90/70	78	16	100	15.5	18	2 +	200	100 molar lactate	100	+150	45	1.023	5.5	9.9	Digoxin 0.25 mg IV push
6:00	86/60	84	16	101.2	14	17	2 + left 3 + right	100		150	+100	40	1.03	5.7	9.3	PO2 105.6 ph 7.56 PCO2 35 O2 sat. 97.8
7:00	86/60	80	16	102.5	14	17	3 +			75	+25	35	1.03	6	9.8	Hypothermia on
8:00	100/60	76	16	101.8	14.5	17	3 +		100 molar lactate	50	-25	30	1.03	6	9.9	MS 3 mg IV
9:00	100/76	76	16	100	12	16	3 +				-25	35	1.03	6	10	Hypothermia off
10:00	100/80	80	16	100	12	16	3 +		100 molar lactate	25	-50	35	1.026	6.5	10	PO2 96 ph 7.58 PCO2 30 O2 sat 97.5
11:00	104/84	84	16	100.2	13	17	3 +				-50	30	1.025	6.5	9	Engstrom changed 5.5 O2 3.5 Air
								500cc		550 cc		405				
									500 cc							
12:00	108/90	86	16	100.6	13	17	3 +		100 molar lactate		-50	35	1.026	6.7	9	MS 3 mg IV Aspirin gr x rectally

271

GLOSSARY

aberrance—a deviation from the usual pattern. In EKG, the temporary abnormal intraventricular conduction of a supraventricular impulse

Adams-Stokes syndrome—a syndrome of loss of consciousness which may be accompanied by convulsions, caused by low cardiac output from a block in AV conduction

akinetic—pertaining to lack of movement or paralysis

anasarca—generalized edema following an increase in interstitial fluid of the body

aneurysm—a dilatation of a section of a blood vessel to form a sac

angina pectoris—a clinical term for a condition caused by disease of the coronary arteries. The usual symptoms are paroxysmal pain accompanied by a sense of constriction about the chest and by indigestion

angiocardiography—x-ray examination of the heart and blood vessels that have been made opaque by injection of a radiopaque media

anoxia—an inadequate oxygen supply to the tissues

antagonism—interaction of two agents in which one agent nullifies the action of the other

anticoagulant—an agent that delays blood clotting

apnea—cessation of breathing

apneustic—exaggerated inspiratory activity without expiration

arteriography—x-ray examination of an artery that has been made opaque by injection of radiopaque media

arteriosclerosis—a condition of the arteries characterized by narrowing of the lumen and loss of elasticity

ascites—a collection of serous fluid in the abdomen

atelectasis—inability to expand the alveoli of the lung from a collapsed state

atherosclerosis—a degenerative process of the arteries characterized by deposits of lipids, salts, and fibrous tissues beneath the intima

auscultation—the process of listening for sounds within the body, usually with a stethoscope

ballistocardiogram—a tracing of the recoil movements of the body caused by the beating of the heart; may be used to calculate cardiac output

baroreceptor—a nerve terminal that is stimulated by changes in pressure

blood pressure—the force exerted by the blood against the blood vessel wall

bradycardia—abnormally slow heart rate

bradypnea—a slow respiratory rate

bronchospasm—spasmodic narrowing of the bronchi

Cannon wave—a large positive jugular venous pulse wave produced by atrial contraction against the closed tricuspid valve of ventricular systole. In ventricular tachycardia, irregularly occurring Cannon waves are of diagnostic value, since they indicate AV dissociation

capillaries—the network of vessels between the arterioles and the veins. Oxygen and nutritive materials diffuse through the walls into the tissues and carbon dioxide and waste products from the tissues enter the circulatory system

cardiac cycle—the heart activity from the initiation of the impulse for depolarization to the completion of repolarization

cardiac output—the volume of blood pumped by the left ventricle of the heart per minute

cardiac tamponade—compression of the heart caused by a collection of fluid in the pericardial sac

cardiotonic—a substance that stimulates the heart to improve its muscular tension

cardioversion—the procedure of delivering a countershock to the heart that is programmed to occur after the impulse for depolarization has spread across the atrium. The purpose is to interrupt an abnormal rhythm so that the normal rhythm can take over

carotid sinus (or body)—a collection of vagal cells near the bifurcation of the carotid artery that are sensitive to pressure and carbon dioxide content of the blood. Massage of these bodies stimulates the vagus and may slow the atrial heart rate

catecholamines—secretions of the adrenal glands that have an adrenergic effect of increasing the blood pressure, heart rate, and perspiration

chemorecptor—a receptor sensitive to chemical changes in the circulating blood, such as a decrease in oxygen tension

cholesterol—a crystalline substance found in animal fat and oil

chordae tendineae—tendinous cords that join the papillary muscles of the heart with the valves

chronotropic—affecting the rate of muscular contraction

cineangiography—a part of the process of cardiac catheterization and angiography that utilizes frames taken at a rapid rate to show movement of the structures and contrast media

claudication—weakness of the legs accompanied by cramplike pains in the calves caused by poor circulation of the blood to the legs

colloid—the dissolved proteins of the plasma and interstitial fluids

congener—a member of the same family, with a common action, effect, or function

cor pulmonale—right ventricular failure resulting from pulmonary disease with pulmonary hypertension crepitation—a crackling feeling or sound commonly used to describe the condition that results when air escapes into the tissues

cyanosis—a bluish coloration of the skin and mucous membranes that accompanies inadequate oxygenation of the blood to the tissues

defibrillator—a machine used to deliver an electrical charge to the heart. Also termed a depolarizer

depolarization—discharge of electrical impulse or neutralization of polarity

diastole—period of relaxation of the heart

dicrotic notch—the depression in the peripheral arterial pressure wave caused by the closing of the aortic valve. It occurs before the second elevation that is produced by the reflected waves from the periphery

digitalization—the process of administering a digitalis drug until the physiological effect is produced

diuretic—a product that increases the output of urine by the kidneys

dyspnea—difficult or labored breathing

ecchymosis—an extravasation of blood under the skin

ectopic—an impulse for heart depolarization that is initiated by a focus other than the sinoatrial node

edema—an abnormally large collection of fluid in the intercellular tissues

electrocardiogram—a graphic tracing of the electrical activity of the heart

electrode—a contact for introduction or detection of electrical activity

electrolyte—a substance that dissociates in water into electrically charged particles capable of conducting an electrical current

embolus—an abnormal material in the blood stream that may lodge in some vessel and obstruct the circulation to the area served by the vessel

emphysema of the lung—a condition in which the alveoli become distended and destroyed

encephalomalacia—softening of the brain from a deficient blood supply, which may be the result of an embolus

endarterectomy—the surgical removal of atheromatous material from the intima of an artery

enzyme—a substance that is capable of initiating or accelerating certain biochemical processes in the body

exsanguination—the forceful loss of blood

extension—an exercise that involves straightening a bent joint

extracorporeal circulation—circulation that takes place outside the body, as by the use of a mechanical pump and oxygenator

extrasystole—a contraction of the heart that is not part of the normal rhythm

fibrillation—twitching or quivering of the muscle cells

fibrin—the insoluble protein of a blood clot

fibrinogen—a soluble protein in the blood plasma which, by the action of thrombin, is converted into fibrin

fibrinogenemia—a condition in which there is an excessive amount of fibrinogen in the blood

fibrinolytic—an agent that has the ability to dissolve a blood clot

flexion—an exercise that involves bending a joint

gallop rhythm—an extra heart sound that resembles a horse's gallop when the heart rate is fast heart block—an interruption in the conduction of the electrical impulse through the atrioventricular node

hematocrit—the volume percentage of red cells in the blood

hemodynamics—the study of the factors affecting the flow and the force of the circulating blood

hemoglobinuria—the presence of hemoglobin in the urine

hemolysis—alteration or destruction of the blood cells

hemopericardium—a collection of blood within the pericardial sac

hemothorax—an accumulation of blood within the thorax, usually in the pleural cavity

hepatization—a change in tissue in which it develops the appearance of liver tissue

hepatomegaly—enlargement of the liver

Hoffman's sign (digital reflex)—sudden flexion of the terminal phalanx of the thumb and second and third phalanges of some other finger elicited by snapping the terminal phalanx of the patient's middle or index finger

homeostasis—the process of maintaining equilibrium

homograft—a transplant of tissue or a graft from one member of a species to another member of the same species

homologous—corresponding in type, structure, and origin

hydrostatic pressure—the pressure exerted by the weight of the column of fluid extending from the heart to any given point of measurement

hypercapnia—an increase in the carbon dioxide content

hypercarbia—an abnormally high level of carbon dioxide in the blood

hyperglycemia—an increase in the amount of glucose in the blood above 100 mg per 100 ml

hyperkalemia—elevation of potassium level in the blood serum above 5.5 mEq/liter

hypernatremia—elevation of the sodium in the blood serum above 145 mEq/liter

hyperosmolarity—the property of having a greater concentration of solutes than the comparison substance

hyperpnea—increased respiratory rate and depth

hypertension—elevation of blood pressure above the normal range

hypertrophy—enlargement of a tissue or organ

hypervolemia—an increase above normal in the volume of circulating blood

hypocapnia—a decreased level of carbon dioxide in the blood

hypochloremia—decrease in the chloride in the blood serum below 95 mEq/liter

hypoglycemia—abnormally low blood sugar (less than 60 mg per 100 ml true glucose)

hypokalemia—decrease in the level of potassium in the blood serum below 3.5 mEq/liter

hyponatremia—a decrease in the sodium in the blood serum below 135 mEq/liter

hypotension—blood pressure below the normal range

hypothermia—the lowering of the body temperature below normal

hypovolemia—a decrease below normal in the volume of circulating blood

hypoxemia—low oxygen tension of the blood

hypoxia—deficiency of oxygen in the inspired air

iatrogenic—occurring as a result of medical or surgical treatment

idiopathic—cause of condition is unknown

idioventricular—originating in the ventricle

incompetent valve—a valve that does not close completely, allowing a backflow of blood. Also called valvular insufficiency

infarct—an area of tissue death caused by lack of adequate blood supply

inotropic—affecting the force of muscular contractions

inspissation—the process of becoming dry or thick by evaporation

interstitial—the area between the cells and the intravascular area

intima—the endothelium that lines the blood vessels

ischemia—insufficient blood supply to an area to maintain normal muscle function

isoelectric—the electrical baseline in an electrocardiogram in which no electrical force is present

Kussmaul respiration—a specific type of rapid, deep, forceful respiration

labile—subject to much variation

lumen—the passageway inside a blood vessel or other tubular organ

mean pressure—the average blood pressure throughout the cardiac cycle. It is determined by taking the diastolic pressure plus one-third of the pulse pressure

metabolic acidosis—a deficiency of base bicarbonate ions that results in a lowered capacity of the blood for buffering and an excessive hydrogen-ion concentration in the body fluids with a decrease in plasma pH below 7.35

metabolic alkalosis—an excessive concentration of base bicarbonate ions with a deficit of hydrogen ions in the body fluids that results in an increase of the plasma pH above 7.45

metabolism—the sum of the physical and chemical changes that occur within the body

mucolytic—tending to dissolve or liquefy mucus

mural thrombus—a blood clot originating from a diseased area of the endocardium

murmur—an abnormal heart sound

myocardium—the muscular wall of the heart that lies between the endocardium on the inside of the heart and the epicardium on the outside of the heart

necrosis—tissue death

neurocirculatory asthenia—a syndrome of nervous and circulary symptoms that does not result from organic disease

occlusion—obstruction of flow through a vessel

oliguria—a diminution in urine output in relation to fluid intake

oncotic pressure—the osmotic pressure that is generated by the colloids at the capillary membrane

orthopnea—condition in which the erect position is necessary for adequate ventilation

osmolality—an expression of the concentration of a solute per unit of solvent

osmolarity—an expression of the concentration of a solute per unit of total volume of the solution

osmoreceptors—nerve receptors that are sensitive to changes in fluid tonicity

osmosis—the phenomenon of the passage of fluid from an area of lesser concentration to an area of greater concentration

P wave—the portion of the electrical recording of the activity of the heart that is produced by the spread of the impulse for contraction across the atria

pacemaker—that area, organ, or instrument that initiates the impulse for heart depolarization

palpation—the process of examining by feeling with the hand

palpitation—a fluttering or rapid pulsation of the heart that can be felt by the person

papillary muscles—muscle fibers in the ventricular walls to which the chordae tendineae are attached

paradoxical pulse—pulse that decreases or disappears during inspiration

partial pressure—the pressure exerted by a specific gas in a mixture of gases

passive exercise—exertion of a body part of a patient without the participation of the patient

patency—a condition of being freely open

perfusion—the passage of a fluid, especially the passage of blood, through the vessels of an organ or area

pericardicentesis—surgical aspiration of fluid from the pericardial sac

pericardium—the double-layered sac enclosing the heart

peripheral resistance—the resistance to the flow of blood that is determined by the tone of the muscles and the diameter of the vessels

peritoneal dialysis—use of the peritoneum as a semipermeable membrane for the removal of desired solutes from the body

phlebitis—inflammation of a vein

phonocardiogram—a graphic recording of heart sounds

pneumothorax—an accumulation of air in the pleural cavity which may result in collapse of the lung

polarity—the property of having an electric potential or charge

potentiate—to increase the acitivity of an agent

P-R interval—that portion of the electrical recording of the activity of the heart that represents the spread of the electrical impulse across the atria and through the AV node

precordium—the area of the chest that is over the heart

pulse—the expansion and contraction of an artery

pulse deficit—the difference between the heart and the peripheral pulse rate

pulse pressure—the difference between the systolic and the diastolic blood pressure

pulsus alternans—a pulse characterized by alternating strong and weak pulsations

Purkinje fibers—specialized muscle fibers found throughout the walls of the ventricles that conduct the impulse for depolarization

QRS complex—that portion of the recorded electrical activity of the heart that is produced by depolarization of the ventricles

Q-T interval—the period on the record of electrical activity from the onset of depolarization to the end of repolarization

rale—an abnormal breath sound caused by some degree of obstruction to the flow of air

refractory—resistant

repolarization—the restoration of polarity or the ability to conduct an electrical current

respiratory acidosis—inadequate pulmonary ventilation with retention of carbon dioxide and an increase in carbonic acid respiratory alkalosis—a decrease in the carbonic acid concentration of the extracellular fluid caused by hyperventilation, which blows off carbon dioxide

reticuloendothelial system—a network of cells concerned primarily with resistance to infection (by their phagocytic action) and blood cell formation

retrograde—to travel in a reverse direction

rheologic agent—an agent that affects the flow of matter, such as the flow of blood through the heart and blood vessels

rouleaux—a group of red blood corpuscles whose formation resembles a pile of coins

septicemia—active bacterial infection of the blood stream

serotonin—a vasoactive substance released from certain tissue cells with a strong epinephrine activity

shock—a state of inadequate tissue perfusion that results from a decreased effective circulating blood volume

shock lung—a syndrome of pulmonary insufficiency following shock

shunt—a diversion

sinus rhythm—heart rhythm that is initiated in the SA node

S-T segment—that portion of the record of electrical activity of the heart from the end of ventricular depolarization to the beginning of repolarization

stenosis—a narrowing or constriction of an opening

stroke volume—the amount of blood ejected with each contraction of the left ventricle

surfactant—a complex lipoprotein secreted by the alveoli which changes its surface tension with changes in the alveolar dimensions, to prevent the alveoli from collapsing completely

sympatholytic—a substance that blocks the impulses conveyed by the adrenergic postganglionic fibers of the sympathetic nervous system

sympathomimetic—a substance that produces an effect similar to stimulation of the adrenergic postganglionic fibers of the sympathetic nervous system

syncope—a sudden but transient loss of consciousness caused by inadequate cerebral flow

syndrome—a group of symptoms that occur together and are given a name to identify the specific combination of symptoms

synergism—interaction of two agents that results in an exaggerated effect of both agents

systole—the period of contraction of the heart

T wave—that period of the recording of the electrical activity of the heart that represents ventricular repolarization

tachycardia—a rapid heart rate over 100 beats per minute

tachypnea—rapid and shallow respiration

thrombin—an enzyme in the blood derived from prothrombin that is responsible for the conversion of fibrinogen into fibrin

thrombolytic—causing the dissolution of a blood clot

thrombophlebitis—the accumulation of a blood clot within a vein accompanied by inflammation

thrombus—a blood clot inside a blood vessel or chamber of the heart that remains at the place of its formation

toxicity—harmful quality

turgor—normal cellular tension or fullness

U wave—an occasionally appearing deflection in the recorded electrical activity of the heart that follows the T wave

vagolytic—a substance that blocks or depresses the impulses conveyed by the vagus nerves

vagotonic—a substance that produces an effect similar to stimulation of the vagus nerve

Valsalva maneuver—a forceful expiratory effort against a closed glottis

valvular insufficiency—inadequate or incompetent closure of a valve which permits a backflow of blood in the wrong direction

vasoconstrictor—an agent that decreases the diameter of blood vessels by producing contraction of the smooth muscles in the walls of the vessels

vasodilator—an agent that increases the diameter of blood vessels by producing relaxation of the smooth muscles in the walls of the vessels

vasopressor—a vasoconstrictor substance that causes the muscles of the arteries to contract

vectorcardiography—determination of the direction and magnitude of the electrical forces of the heart

REFERENCES

1. Swan, H. J.: Complications of Cardiac Catheterization, *Cardio-Vascular Nursing*, 4:6: 27–30 (1968).

2. Braunwald, E. and H. J. Swan: Cooperative Study on Cardiac Catheterization, *Circulation*, 37–38 (suppl. 3):17–26 (1968).

3. Kaplan, S. M.: Psychological Aspects of Cardiac Disease, *Psychosomatic Medicine*, 18:233 (March 1956).

4. Brambilla, M. A.: An Investigation of Patients' Questions about Heart Surgery: Implications for Nursing, "ANA Clinical Sessions," Appleton-Century-Crofts, New York, 1968, pp. 217–222.

5. Bartlett, Robert M.: Post-Traumatic Pulmonary Insufficiency, "Surgery Annual," Appleton-Century-Crofts, New York, Vol. 3, 1971.

6. Doyle, J. T. et al.: The Relationship of Cigarette Smoking to Coronary Heart Disease, *J.A.M.A.*, 190:886–890 (1964).

7. McGoon, D. C.: Techniques of Open-Heart Surgery for Congenital Heart Disease, *Current Problems in Surgery*, April 1968.

8. Sonnenblick, E. H.: Correlation of Myocardial Ultrastructure and Function, *Circulation*, 38:29 (1968).

9. Sirak, H. D.: "Operable Heart Disease, Pathophysiology, Diagnosis, and Treatment," C.V. Mosby Co., St. Louis, 1966.

10. Blair, E.: "Clinical Hypothermia," McGraw-Hill Book Company, New York, 1964.

11. Neville, W. E.: Extracorporeal Circulation, *Current Problems in Surgery*, July 1967.

12. Thal, A. P. and R. F. Wilson: Shock, *Current Problems in Surgery*, September 1965.

13.	Lane, C.: Intra-Aortic Phase Shift Balloon Pumping in Cardiogenic Shock, *Am. J. Nurs.*, **69**:1655–1659 (1969).

14.	Buckley, M. J. et al.: Hemodynamic Evaluation of Intra-Aortic Balloon Pumping in Man, *Circulation*, **42**(suppl. 2):130–134 (1970).

15.	Hirai, J., A. Wakabayashi, and J. E. Connolly: A New Method of Pulsatile Bypass Without Heparin for Aortic Arch Replacement, *Trans. Amer. Soc. Artif. Int. Organs*, **27**:183–186 (1971).

16.	Wakabayashi, A., J. Hirai, E. Stemmer, and J. Connolly: Heparinless Total Left Heart Bypass with induced Ventricular Fibrillation, *Am. J. Surg.*, **122**:2:243–248 (1971).

17.	Crandell, Walter B.: Parenteral Fluid Therapy, *Surg. Clin. North America*, **48**:4:707–721 (1968).

18.	Gauer, D. H., J. R. Henry, and H. Sieker: Cardiac Receptors and Fluid Volume Control, *Prog. Cardiovas. Diseases*, **4**:1–26 (1961).

19.	Zimmerman, B.: Postoperative Management of Fluid Volumes and Electrolytes, *Current Problems in Surgery*, December 1965.

20.	Shires, T., J. Williams, and R. Brown: Acute Changes in Extracellular Fluids Associated with Major Surgical Procedures, *Ann. Surg.*, **154**:803–810 (1961).

21.	Marks, L. J., R. B. Gibson, and H. Oyama: Effect of Preoperative Isotonic Expansion of Extracellular Fluid Volume on Postoperative Renal Sodium Excretion, *Surgery*, **54**:456–462 (1963).

22.	Krohn, B. G., R. R. Urquhart, O. Magidson, H. Tsuji, J. V. Redington, and J. H. Kay: Metabolic Alkalosis Following Heart Surgery, *J. Thoracic Cardiovas. Surg.*, **56**:5:732–747 (1968).

23.	Crandell, Walter B.: The Relation of Excessive Intravenous Fluid Administration to Postoperative Mortality, *Trans. New England Surg. Soc.*, **41**:139–151 (1960).

24.	Dudrick, S. J., D. W. Wilmore, H. M. Vars, and J. E. Rhodes: Long-Term Total Parenteral Nutrition with Growth, Development, and Positive Nitrogen Balance, *Surgery*, **64**:134–142 (1968).

25.	Shires, G. T. and C. R. Baxter: Complications of Parenteral Fluid Therapy, in C. P. Artz, and J. D. Hardy, (eds.), "Complications in Surgery and Their Management," W. B. Saunders Company, Philadelphia and London, 1967, pp. 68–80.

26.	Collins, R. et al.: Risk of Local and Systemic Infection with Polyethylene Intravenous Catheters, *New England J. Med.*, **279**:340 (1968).

27.	Bentley, D. W. and M. H. Lepper: Septicemia Related to Indwelling Venous Catheters, *J.A.M.A.*, **206**:1759 (1968).

28.	Hoshal, V. L. et al.: Fibrin Sleeve Formation on Indwelling Subclavian Central Venous Catheters, *Arch. Surg.*, **102**:353–358 (1971).

29.	Ayres, S. A. and S. Giannelli: "Care of the Critically Ill," Appleton-Century-Crofts, New York, 1969.

30.	Comroe, Julius H.: "Physiology of Respiration," Year Book Medical Publishers, Inc., Chicago, 1965.

31.	Moseley, R. V. and D. B. Doty: Changes in the Filtration Characteristics of Stored Blood, *Ann. Surg.*, **171**:329 (1970).

32.	Clements, John: Surface Active Materials in the Lung, in Liebow, A. A., and Smith, D. F. (eds.), "The Lung," Williams and Wilkins Co., Baltimore, 1968, pp. 31–39.

33.	Gazzaniga, A. B. and N. E. O'Conner: The Effects of Intravenous Infusion of Autologous Kidney Lysosomal Enzymes in the Dog, *Ann. Surg.*, **172**:804–812 (1970)

34.	Blaisdell, R. W., R. C. Lim, Jr., and R. J. Stallone: The Mechanism of Pulmonary Damage Following Traumatic Shock, *Surg. Gynec. & Obstet.*, **130**:15 (1970).

35. Bendixen, H., J. Hedley-Whyte, and M. B. Laver: Impaired Oxygenation in Surgical Patients During General Anesthesia with Controlled Ventilation. A Concept of Atelectasis, *New England J. Med.*, **269**:991–996 (1963).

36. Stemmer, E. A., J. E. Connolly, and J. Kwann: The Role of Blood Gas Determinations in Postoperative Management, presented at the So. Calif. Chapter of American College of Surgeons, San Diego, Calif., January 18, 1960.

37. Ayres, Larry: Oxygen Toxicity, *Current Concepts in Chest Diseases*, **11**:1 (1971).

38. Christlieb, I. I., J. F. Dammann, Jr., N. S. Thung, and W. H. Muller: Postoperative Care in Surgery: A Frequent Determinant of Success or Failure, *Dis. Chest*, **44**:1 (1963).

39. ———, ———, and ———: Blood CO_2 Measured Through Skin, *J.A.M.A.*, **205**:19–20 (1968).

40. Maloney, J. V. et al.: Electrophrenic Respiration. Comparison of Effects of Positive Pressure Breathing and Electrophrenic Respiration on the Circulation During Hemorrhagic Shock and Barbiturate Poisoning, *Surg. Gynec. & Obstet.*, **92**:672–684 (1951).

41. Thung, N., Herzog, I. I. Christlieb, W. M. Thompson, and J. F. Dammann, Jr.: The Cost of Respiratory Effort in Postoperative Cardiac Patients, *Circulation*, **28**:552–559 (1963).

42. Baxter, W. D. and R. S. Levine: An Evaluation of Intermittent Positive Pressure Breathing in the Prevention of Postoperative Pulmonary Complications, *Arch. Surg.*, **98**:795 (1969).

43. Mahoney, P. D. and F. J. Calgan: The Effect of Dead Space Rebreathing in the Treatment of Atelectasis, *Surg. Gynec. & Obstet.*, **128**:1283 (1969).

44. Bartlett, R. H., P. Krop, L. Hanson, and F. D. Moore: The Physiology of Yawning and Its Application to Postoperative Care, *Surg. Forum*, **21**:222 (1970).

45. Didier, Edward P. and A. A. Sessler: Postoperative Respiratory Failure, *Surg. Clin. North America*, **49**:5 (1969).

46. Kurihara, M.: Postural Drainage, Clapping, and Vibrating, *Am. J. Nurs.*, **65**:11:76–79 (1965).

47. Strand, F. L.: "Modern Physiology," The Macmillan Company, New York, 1965.

48. Wilson, J. M., J. B. Grow, C. V. Demong, A. E. Prevedel, and J. C. Owens: Central Venous Pressure in Optimal Blood Volume Maintenance, *Arch Surg.*, **85**:4:563–578 (1962).

49. Collins, J. A. and W. F. Ballinger: The Surgical Intensive Care Unit, *Surgery*, **66**:614–619 (1969).

50. Ahlquist, R. P.: A Study of the Adrenotropic Receptors, *Am. J. Physiol.*, **153**:586–600 (1948).

51. Bellet, S. and J. Kostis: Study of Cardiac Arrhythmias by Ultrasonic Doppler Method, *J.A.M.A.*, **204**:530 (1968).

52. Marriott, H. J. L.: "Practical Electrocardiography," Waverly Press, Inc., Baltimore, Md., 1968.

53. Bull, J. P.: Circulatory Responses to Blood Loss and Injury, in Allgower, M. (ed), "Progress in Surgery," Hafner Publishing Co., New York, 1964.

54. Fishman, N. H., J. C. Hutchinson, and B. B. Roe: Controlled

Atrial Hypertension: A Method for Supporting Cardiac Output Following Open-Heart Surgery, *J. Thoracic and Cardiovas. Surg.*, **52**:6 (1966).

55. Fishman, N. H., B. B. Roe, A. Benson, and J. Hutchinson: Control of the Hazards of Cardiac Valve Replacement, *Am. J. Surg.*, **112**:218 (1966).

56. Joly, H. and M. Weil: Temperature of the Great Toe as an Indication of the Severity of Shock, *Circulation*, **35**:131–138 (1969).

57. Marriott, H. J. L. and E. Fogg: Constant Monitoring for Cardiac Dysrhythmias and Blocks, *Modern Concepts of Cardiovascular Disease* **39**:6:103–108 (1970).

58. Olson, E. V.: Immobility. Effects on Cardiovascular Function, *Am. J. Nurs.*, **67**:4:781–787 (1967).

59. Halpern, A., N. Shaftel, D. Selman, and H. Birch: The Cardiovascular Dynamics of Bowel Function, *Angiology*, **9**:99–111 (1958).

60. DuBois, E. F.: "Fever and the Regulation of Body Temperature," Charles C Thomas, Springfield, Ill., 1948.

61. Weil, M. H. and H. Shubin: A VIP Approach to Shock, *J.A.M.A.*, **207**:337 (1969).

62. Chazan, J. W., R. Stenson, and G. S. Kurland: The Acidosis of Cardiac Arrest, *New England J. Med.*, **278**:360–364 (1968).

63. Vaughn, C. C., H. R. Warner, and R. M. Nelson: Cardiovascular Effects of Glucagon Following Cardiac Surgery, *Surgery*, **67**:1:204–211 (January 1970).

64. Yokes, J. A. and W. A. Reed: Heart Surgery, in Meltzer, L. A., Abdellah, F. G., and Kitchell, R. J. (eds.), "Concepts and Practices for Intensive Care," The Charles Press, Philadelphia, 1969, pp. 374–394.

65. Boyan, C. P. and W. S. Howland: Immediate and Delayed Mortality Associated with Massive Blood Transfusions, *Surg. Clin. North America*, **49**:2:217–222 (1969).

66. Stefanini, M. and W. Dameshek: "The Hemorrhagic Disorders," Grune and Stratton, New York, 1962, pp. 510–514.

67. Brunner, L., C. Emerson, L. Ferguson, and D. Suddarth: "Textbook of Medical-Surgical Nursing," J. B. Lippincott Co., Philadelphia, New York, Toronto, 1970.

68. Silver, D. and F. H. McGregor, Jr.: Nonmechanical Causes of Surgical Bleeding, *Current Problems in Surgery* (January 1970).

69. Fine, Jacob: Septic Shock, *J.A.M.A.*, **188**:5:127–132 (1964).

70. Harrison, T. S., R. C. Chawla, and R. S. Wojtalik: Steroidal Influences on Catecholamines, *New England J. Med.*, **279**:136–143 (1968).

71. Conn, J.: Shock, in Beal, J. M. and Eckenhoff, J. (eds.), "Intensive and Recovery Room Care," The Macmillan Co., Collier-Macmillan Ltd., London, 1969, pp. 147–176.

72. Lillehei, R. C. et al.: The Modern Treatment of Shock Based on Physiologic Principles, *Clin. Pharm. & Ther.*, **5**:88–89 (1964).

73. Deterling, R.: Acute Arterial Occlusion, *Surg. Clin. North America*, **46**:3:587–604 (1966).

74. Wheeler, H. B.: Management of Acute Arterial Insufficiency, *Surg. Clin. North America*, **48**:4:851–868 (1968).

75. Meyer, O. O.: Treatment with Anticoagulants, *Cardio-Vascular Nursing*, **4**:3:11–15 (1968).

76. Evarts, C. M.: The Fat Embolism Syndrome, *Arizona Med.*, **26**:155–166 (1969).

77. Wolff, H. G. et al.: Changes in Form and Function of Mucous

Membranes Occurring as Part of Protective Reaction Patterns in Man during Periods of Life Stress and Emotional Conflict, *Trans. Assoc. Am. Physicians*, 61:313 (1948).

78. Dennis, L. B.: "Psychology of Human Behavior for Nurses," W. B. Saunders Company, Philadelphia and London, 1967.

79. Schlesinger, B.: "Higher Cerebral Functions and Their Clinical Disorders," Grune and Stratton, New York, 1962.

80. Solomon, P. et al.: "Sensory Deprivation," Harvard University Press, Cambridge, Mass., 1961.

81. Kornfeld, D. S., S. Zimberg, and J. Malm: Psychiatric Complications of Open-Heart Surgery, *New England J. Med.*, 273:287–292 (1965).

82. Blachly, P. H. and A. Starr: Post-Cardiotomy Delirium, *Am. J. Psychiat.*, 121:371–375 (1964).

83. Krystal, H.: The Physiological Basis of the Treatment of Delirium Tremens, *Am. J. Psychiat.*, 116:137–147 (1959).

84. Liberson, W. T.: Electroencephalography, *Am. J. Psychiat.*, 116:584 (1960).

85. Jourard, S. M.: "The Transparent Self," D. Van Nostrand Co., Inc., Princeton, N. J. 1964.

86. Turner, R.: Role-Taking, Role Standpoint, and Reference Group Behavior, *Am. J. Sociol.* 61:316–328 (1956).

87. Nite, G. and F. Willis: "The Coronary Patient—Hospital Care and Rehabilitation," The Macmillan Co., New York, 1964.

88. Hamburg, D. A., B. Hamburg, and S. de Goza: Adaptive Problems in Severely Burned Patients, *Psychiatry*, 16:1–20 (February 1953).

89. Brown, E. L.: "Newer Dimensions of Patient Care. Part II," Russell Sage Foundation, New York, 1964.

90. Van Slyke, K. K. and E. I. Evans: Paradox of Aciduria in the Presence of Hypochloremia, *Ann. Surg.*, 126:545 (1947).

91. Krohn, B. G., O. Magidson, R. R. Lewis, H. Tsuji, J. V. Redington, and J. H. Kay: Prevention of Metabolic Alkalosis Following Heart Surgery, *J. Thoracic and Cardiovas. Surg.*, 56:748 (1968).

92. Kay, J. H., S. Bernstein, H. Tsuji, J. V. Redington, M. Milgram, and T. Brem: Surgical Treatment of Candida Endocarditis, *J.A.M.A.*, 203:621–626 (1968).

93. Engleman, R. M., F. C. Spencer, G. E. Reed, and D. A. Tice: Cardiac Tamponade Following Open-Heart Surgery, *Circulation*, 42 (suppl. 2): 165–171 (1970).

94. Merrill, J. P.: Acute Renal Failure, *J.A.M.A.*, 211:289–291 (1970).

95. Powers, S. R., J. E. Kiley, and A. Boba: Renal Failure in Surgical Patients, *Current Problems in Surgery* (November 1964).

96. ——, ——, and ——: Pain, Part I: Basic Concepts and Assessment (Programmed Instruction Supplement), *Am. J. Nurs.*, 66:1085–1108 (1966).

97. Blaylock, J: The Psychological and Cultural Influences on the Reaction to Pain, *Nurs. Forum*, 7:262–274 (1968).

98. Petrie, A.,T. Holland, and I. Wolk: "Perceptual Indicators of Basic Algesic Types—A New Look at Pain and Suffering," Briefs, Maternity Center Association, 26:8, New York (October 1962).

99. McCaffery, M. and M. Moss: Nursing Intervention for Bodily Pain, *Am. J. Nurs.*, 67:6:1224–1227 (1967).

100. Boyar, J. I. and E. P. Gramlich: Unusual Postsurgical Pain, *Surg. Clin. North America*, 50:2:309–318 (April 1970).

101. Holley, H. S.: Immediate Postoperative Management, in Beal, J. M. and Eckenhoff, J. E. (eds.), "Intensive and Recovery Room Care," The Macmillan Company, Collier-Macmillan Ltd., London, 1969, pp. 53–70.

102. Janis, I. L.: "Psychological Stress," John Wiley and Sons, New York, 1958.

103. Moss, E. T. and B. Meyers: Effect of Nursing Intervention upon Pain Relief in Patients, *Nurs. Res.*, **15**:303–306 (1966).

104. Parsons, T.: "The Social System," The Free Press, Glencoe, Ill., 1951.

105. Allen, W. H.: "Indications for Intravenous Pacers," presented at the Instrumental Acquisition of Cardiological Data, Long Beach, Calif., August 1968.

106. Braunwald, N. S., W. A. Gay, Jr., A. G. Morrow, and E. Braunwald: Sustained, Paired Electrical Stimuli, *Am. J. Card.*, **14**:385–393 (July–December 1964).

107. Iseri, L. T.: "Percutaneous Pacing," presented at the Instrumental Acquisition of Cardiological Data, Long Beach, Calif., August 1968.

108. Spandau, M.: Insertion of Temporary Cardiac Pacemakers Without Fluoroscopy, *Am. J. Nurs.*, **70**:1011–1013 (May 1970).

109. Furman, S. et al.: Implanted Transvenous Pacemakers: Equipment, Technique, and Clinical Experience, *Ann. Surg.*, **164**:465–474 (1966).

110. Calvin, J. W., E. A. Stemmer, R. A. Steedman, and J. E. Connolly: Clinical Application of Parasternal Mediastinotomy, *Arch. Surg.*, **102**:322–325 (1971).

111. ———, ———, ———, and ———: "Cardiovascular Surgery," U.S. Dept. of Health, Education, and Welfare, Washington, D. C., 1968.

112. Williams, G. D. and G. S. Campbell: Long-term Management of Cardiac Pacemakers with a Systematic Approach to Malfunction, *Surgery*, **66**:644–654 (1969).

113. Center, Sol: "Evaluation of Pacemaker Dysfunction," presented at the Instrumental Acquisition of Cardiological Data, Long Beach, Calif., August 1968.

114. Walker, W. J.: "Electrolytes and Their Influence on Pacing," presented at the Instrumental Acquisition of Cardiological Data, Long Beach, Calif., August 1968.

115. Olson, E. V.: Closed Chest Cardiopulmonary Resuscitation, *Cardio-Vascular Nursing*, **2**:2:23–26 (1966).

116. Grace, W. J.: Detection and Treatment of Cardiac Arrhythmias by Electrical Means, in Ayres, S. And Gianelli, S. (eds.), "Care of the Critically Ill," Appleton-Century-Crofts, New York 1967, pp. 195–206.

117. ———: Cardiopulmonary Resuscitation, Statement by the Ad Hoc Committee on Cardiopulmonary Resuscitation of the Division of Medical Sciences, National Academy of Sciences–National Research Council, *J.A.M.A.*, **198**:4:372–379 (1966).

118. Gildea, J. E.: Cardiovascular Resuscitation, in Beal, J. M. and Eckenhoff, J. E. (eds.), "Intensive and Recovery Room Care," The Macmillan Co., New York, 1969, pp. 122–142.

119. Jude, J. R. and O. J. Elam: "Fundamentals of Cardiovascular Resuscitation," F. A. Davis Co., Philadelphia, 1965.

120. Kreel, Isadore et al.: A Syndrome Following Total Body Perfusion, *Surg. Gynec. & Obstet.*, **111**:317 (1960).

121. Pirofsky, B.: Hemolysis in Valvular Heart Disease, *Ann Int. Med.*, **65**:373 (1966).

122. Cooley, M. H.: Intravascular Hemolysis Syndrome Following Aortic Valve Replacement, *Arch. Int. Med.*, **118**:486 (1966).

123. Griepp, R. B., E. B. Stinson, D. A. Clark, and N. E. Shumway: A Two-Year Experience with Human Heart Transplantation, *California Med.*, **113**:17–26 (August 1970).

124. Shumway, N. E., E. Dong, and E. Stinson: "Surgical Aspects of Cardiac Transplantations in Man," Symposium on Surgical, Immunological, and Ethical Transplantations in Man, New York, May 10, 1968.

125. Stinson, E. B., E. Dong, W. Angell, and N. Shumway: Myocardia Hypothermia for Cardiac Transplantation, *Laval Medical*, **41**:2:195–198 (1970).

126. Griepp, R., E. Stinson, E. Dong, D. Clark, and N. Shumway: Determinants of Operative Risk in Human Heart Transplantation, *Am. J. Surg.*, **122**:192–198 (August 1971).

127. Stinson, E. B., E. Dong, C. Bieber, J. Schroeder, and N. Shumway: Cardiac Transplantation in Man, *J.A.M.A.*, **207**:12:2233–2242 (1969).

128. Chartrand, C., W. W. Angell, E. Dong, and N. E. Shumway: Atrial Pacing in the Postoperative Management of Cardiac Homotransplantation, *Ann. Thoracic Surg.*, **8**:2:152–160 (1969).

129. Friesen, W. G., R. D. Woodson, A. W. Ames, R. R. Herr, A. Starr, and D. G. Kassebaum: A Hemodynamic Comparison of Atrial and Ventricular Pacing in Postoperative Cardiac Surgery Patients, *J. Thoracic. Cardiovas. Surg.*, **55**:271 (1968).

130. ——, ——, ——, ——, ——, and ——: Primary Prevention of the Atherosclerotic Diseases, Report of Inter-Society Commission for Heart Disease Resources, *Circulation*, **42**:A72–A78 (1970).

131. Aronson, M.: How to Help Patients Accept Life-Sustaining Devices, *Med.-Surg. Rev.*, **6**:35–43 (1971).

132. Sprague, H. B.: The Heart and the Law, in Hurst, J. W. and Logue, R. B. (eds.), "The Heart," McGraw-Hill Book Company, New York, pp. 1609–1615.

133. Rambousek, E.: The Third Dimension, in Powers, M. and Storlie, F. (eds.), "The Cardiac Surgery Patient," Collier-Macmillan Ltd., London, 1969, pp. 187–203.

134. Hallin, R., U. S. Page, J. C. Bigelow, and W. R. Sweetman: Revascularization of the Heart. Aorto-Bypass in Sixty-Three Patients, *Am. J. Surg.*, **122**:164–168 (August 1971).

135. MacCannell, K. et al.: Dopamine in the Treatment of Hypotension and Shock, *New England J. Med.*, **275**:1389–1398 (1966).

136. Bacaner, M. G.: Rx of Ventricular Fibrillation and Other Ventricular Arrhythmias with Bretylium Tosylate, *J.A.M.A.*, **204**:529 (1968).

137. Shim, C.: Blocking Heart Block in Suctioning, *Medical World News*, **11**:40A (March 1970).

138. Weibell, F. J. and E. A. Pfeiffer: Seminar on the Safe Use of Electrical Equipment in the Hospital (Course Notes), Western Research Support Center, V.A. Hospital, Sepulveda, Calif., 1971.

BIBLIOGRAPHY

Comroe, Julius H.: "Physiology of Respiration," Year Book Medical Publishers, Inc., Chicago, 1965.

Goodman, Louis S. and Afred Gilman: "The Pharmacological Basis of Therapeutics," The Macmillan Company, New York, 1970.

Guyton, A. C.: "Textbook of Medical Physiology," W. B. Saunders Company, Philadelphia, 1971.

Hurst, J. Willis and R. Bruce Logue: "The Heart," 2d ed., McGraw-Hill Book Company, New York, 1970.

Marriott, H. J. L.: "Practical Electrocardiography," Waverly Press, Baltimore, 1968.

Moidel, Harriet C. and Gladys E. Sorensen: "Nursing Care of the Patient with Medical-Surgical Disorders," McGraw-Hill Book Company, New York 1970.

INDEX